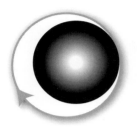

Core
Clinical
Cases in Medicine and Surgery

a problem-solving approach

Edited by

Steve Bain MA MD FRCP
Professor of Medicine (Diabetes), University of Wales,
Swansea & Honorary Consultant Physician, Swansea NHS
Trust, Singleton Hospital, Swansea, UK

Janesh K. Gupta MSC MD FRCOG
Clinical Senior Lecturer/Honorary Consultant in
Obstetrics and Gynaecology, University of Birmingham,
Birmingham Women's Hospital, Birmingham, UK

Core Clinical Cases series edited by

Janesh K. Gupta MSc MD FRCOG
Clinical Senior Lecturer/ Honorary Consultant in
Obstetrics and Gynaecology, University of Birmingham,
Birmingham Women's Hospital, Birmingham, UK

Hodder Arnold
A MEMBER OF THE HODDER HEADLINE GROUP

First published in Great Britain in 2006 by
Hodder Education, a member of the Hodder Headline Group,
338 Euston Road, London NW1 3BH

http://www.hoddereducation.com

Distributed in the United States of America by
Oxford University Press Inc.,
198 Madison Avenue, New York, NY10016
Oxford is a registered trademark of Oxford University Press

British Library Cataloguing in Publication Data
A catalogue record for this book is available from the British Library

Library of Congress Cataloging-in-Publication Data
A catalog record for this book is available from the Library of Congress

ISBN-10: 0 340 81670 8
ISBN-13: 978 0 340 81670 7

1 2 3 4 5 6 7 8 9 10

Commissioning Editor: Georgina Bentliff
Project Editors: Heather Smith and Clare Weber
Production Controller: Jane Lawrence
Cover Design: Georgina Hewitt

Typeset in 9 on 12 pt Frutiger Light Condensed by Phoenix Photosetting, Chatham, Kent
Printed and bound in Malta

What do you think about this book? Or any other Hodder Arnold title?
Please visit our website at www.hoddereducation.com

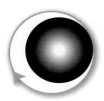

Contents

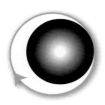

List of contributors

Matthew Clark BHB MBChB MD FRACS, General Surgeon and Clinical Associate Professor of Surgery, University of Auckland, Middlemore Hospital, Auckland, NZ

Indranil Dasgupta MBBS MD DM FRCP, Consultant Nephrologist and Honorary Senior Lecturer, Birmingham Heartlands Hospital, Birmingham, UK

Andrew Levy PhD FRCP, Reader in Medicine, Bristol University, and Honorary Consultant Physician, Bristol Royal Infirmary, Bristol, UK

C. S. Probert MD ILTM FRCP, Consultant and Reader in Gastroenterology, University of Bristol, Department of Clinical Science at South Bristol, Bristol Royal Infirmary, Bristol, UK

Neeraj Prasad MD FRCP, Consultant Cardiologist, Hereford County Hospital, Hereford, UK

Mark Pugh DTM DCH MD FRCPI, Consultant Rheumatologist and Clinical Tutor, Department of Rheumatology, St Mary's Hospital, Newport, Isle of Wight, UK

Malcolm Shepherd MBChB MRCP PhD, Balmforth Intermediate Clinical Scientist Research Fellow, University of Glasgow, Glasgow, UK

Neil C. Thomson MBChB MD FRCP, Professor of Respiratory Medicine, University of Glasgow, Glasgow, UK

Steven Thrush FRCS (Gen Surg), Consultant General Surgeon, Worcester Royal Hospital, Worcester, UK

Nevianna Tomson MBChB MRCP, Specialist Registrar in Dermatology, Addenbrookes' Hospital, Cambridge, UK

Peter Wallis BSc MBBS FRCP, Consultant Geriatrician and Honorary Senior Clinical Lecturer, University of Birmingham, Department of Elderly Medicine, Birmingham Heartlands Hospital, Birmingham, UK

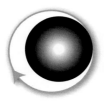

Series preface

'A History Lesson'

Between about 1916 and 1927 a puzzling illness appeared and swept around the world. Dr von Economo first described encephalitis lethargica (EL), which simply meant 'inflammation of the brain that makes you tired'. Younger people, especially women, seemed to be more vulnerable but the disease affected people of all ages. People with EL developed a 'sleep disorder', fever, headache and weakness, which led to a prolonged state of unconsciousness. The EL epidemic occurred during the same time period as the 1918 influenza pandemic, and the two outbreaks have been linked ever since in the medical literature. Some confused it with the epidemic of Spanish flu at that time whereas others blamed weapons used in World War I.

Encephalitis lethargica was dramatized by the film *Awakenings* (book written by Oliver Sacks who is an eminent neurologist from New York), starring Robin Williams and Robert De Niro. Professor Sacks treated his patients with L-dopa, which temporarily awoke his patients, giving rise to the belief that the condition was related to Parkinson's disease.

Since the 1916–27 epidemic, only sporadic cases have been described. Pathological studies have revealed encephalitis of the midbrain and basal ganglia, with lymphocyte (predominantly plasma cell) infiltration. Recent examination of archived EL brain material has failed to demonstrate influenza RNA, adding to the evidence that EL was not an invasive influenza encephalitis. Further investigations found no evidence of viral encephalitis or other recognized causes of rapid-onset parkinsonism. Magnetic resonance imaging (MRI) of the brain was normal in 60 per cent but showed inflammatory changes localized to the deep grey matter in 40 per cent of patients.

As late as the end of the twentieth century, it seemed that the possible answers lay in the clinical presentation of the patients in the 1916–27 epidemic. It had been noted by the clinicians at that time that the central nervous system (CNS) disorder had presented with pharyngitis. This led to the possibility of a post-infectious autoimmune CNS disorder similar to Sydenham's chorea, in which group A β-haemolytic streptococcal antibodies cross-react with the basal ganglia and result in abnormal behaviour and involuntary movements. Anti-streptolysin-O titres have subsequently been found to be elevated in most of these patients. It seemed possible that autoimmune antibodies may cause remitting parkinsonian signs subsequent to streptococcal tonsillitis as part of the spectrum of post-streptococcal CNS disease.

Could it be that the 80-year mystery of EL has been solved relying on the patient's clinical history of presentation, rather than focusing on expensive investigations? More research in this area will give us the definitive answer. This scenario is not dissimilar to the controversy about the idea that streptococcal infections are aetiologically related to rheumatic fever.

With this example of a truly fascinating history lesson, we hope that you will endeavour to use the patient's clinical history as your most powerful diagnostic tool to make the correct diagnosis. If you do you are likely to be right 80–90 per cent of the time. This is the basis of all the Core Clinical Cases series, which will make you systematically explore clinical problems through the clinical history of presentation, followed by examination and the performance of appropriate investigations. Never break that rule.

Janesh Gupta
2006

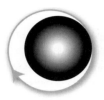

Preface

Why core clinical cases?

In undergraduate medical education there is a trend towards the development of 'core' curricula. The aim is to facilitate the teaching of essential and relevant knowledge, skills and attitudes. This contrasts with traditional medical school courses, where the emphasis was on detailed factual knowledge, often with little obvious clinical relevance. In addition, students' learning is now commonly examined using objective structured clinical examinations (OSCEs) which again assess the practical use of knowledge, rather than the regurgitation of 'small-print'.

Core cases in Medicine and Surgery cannot be an exhaustive list of all of the cases which could be regarded as 'core', largely due to the massive scope of these specialties. However, the volumes do present examples which can be used to train the reader in a realistic way of approaching medical and surgical problems. This should help develop a learning strategy for fifth year medical students to prepare for final examinations, as well as providing useful revision for pre-registration house doctors taking on a new area.

Why a problem-solving approach?

In practice, patients present with clinical problems, which are explored through history, examination and investigation progressively leading from a differential to a definitive diagnosis. Traditionally, textbooks present the subject matter according to a pathophysiological classification which does not help solve real-life clinical scenarios. We have, therefore, based this book on a problem-solving approach. This inculcates the capacity for critical thinking and should help readers to analyse the basis of clinical problems. Of course we accept that the divisions within medicine and surgery are arbitrary, but the areas covered by the specialties are so huge that chapter headings give a steer as to which system will be involved. However, the reader should remember to include other systems in their differential diagnosis, akin to the real life situation where a patient is referred to a neurology clinic with fits but turns out to have a cardiovascular cause for their symptoms.

How will this book inspire problem-solving traits?

The short case scenarios presented in these books are based on common clinical cases which readers are likely to encounter in undergraduate medicine and surgery. These are grouped according to the various subspecialties within medicine and surgery. Groups include varying numbers of cases, each of which begins with a statement of the patient's complaint followed by a short description of the patient's problem. For each case, using a question and short answer format, the reader is taken through a problem-solving exercise.

There are two types of problem-solving cases in this book: one type deals with the development of a diagnostic and therapeutic strategy; whilst the other deals with the development of a counselling strategy. 'Core' information about the subject matter relevant to the patient's problem is also summarized, as this information is helpful for answering the questions. The format of the book enables the cases to be used for learning as well as for self-assessment.

In the cases that deal with diagnostic and therapeutic strategies, the reader is questioned about the interpretation of the relevant clinical features presented, so as to compile an array of likely differential diagnoses. They may then be asked to identify specific pieces of information in the history and to select an appropriate clinical examination which will narrow down the differential list to the most likely diagnosis. This emphasis is important because, in clinical practice, history and examination result in a correct diagnosis in 80–90% of cases. Following this, readers are asked to suggest investigations which would be required to confirm or refute the diagnosis. Once a diagnosis has been reached, readers develop a treatment plan. In general terms, this should first consider conservative non-invasive options (e.g. the important option of doing nothing), followed by medical and surgical options.

In clinical practice, any therapeutic strategy has to be conveyed to patients in a manner that they can understand. Therefore we have included problems that will challenge the reader to develop a counselling strategy. These counselling cases will help and encourage readers to communicate confidently with patients. This generic learning strategy is followed throughout the book with the aim of reinforcing the skills required to master the problem-solving approach.

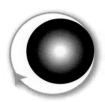

Abbreviations

5-ASA	5-acetylsalicylic acid
AAA	abdominal aortic aneurysm
A&E	accident and emergency
ABGs	arterial blood gases
ABPIs	ankle brachial pressure indices
ACE	angiotensin-converting enzyme
ACR	albumin:creatinine ratio
ACTH	adrenocorticotrophic hormone
AF	atrial fibrillation
Af	atrial flutter
ALI	acute limb ischaemia
ALT	alanine aminotransferase
ALP	alkaline phosphatase
AMR	acute mitral regurgitation
ANA	antinuclear antibody
ANCA	anti-neutrophil cytoplasmic antigen
APD	automated peritoneal dialysis
ARBs	angiotensin II receptor blockers
AR	aortic regurgitation
ARF	acute renal failure
ASD	atrial septal defect
AST	aspartate aminotransferase
ATLS	advanced trauma life support
ATN	acute tubular necrosis
AV	atrioventricular

BAL	bronchoalveolar lavage
BLS	basic life support
BMI	body mass index
BP	blood pressure
BPH	benign prostatic hyperplasia
BTS	British Thoracic Society
CAPD	continuous ambulatory peritoneal dialysis
CCU	coronary care unit
CFA	cryptogenic fibrosing alveolitis
CHD	coronary heart disease
CPK	creatine phosphokinase
CK	creatine kinase
CK-MB	isoenzyme of CK released following myocardial cell damage
CKD	chronic kidney disease
CMV	cytomegalovirus
CNS	central nervous system
COPD	chronic obstructive pulmonary disease
CPAP	continuous positive airway pressure
CPR	cardiopulmonary resuscitation
CRF	chronic renal failure
CRP	C-reactive protein
CSF	cerebrospinal fluid
CT	computed tomography

CTPA	CT pulmonary angiogram		FFP	fresh frozen plasma
CTS	carpal tunnel syndrome		FNA	fine-needle aspiration
CVD	cardiovascular disease		FNAB	fine-needle aspiration biopsy
CVP	central venous pressure		FSGS	focal segmental glomerulosclerosis
CVVH	continuous veno-venous haemofiltration		FSH	follicle-stimulating hormone
DC	direct current		fT$_4$	free thyroxine
DEXA	dual energy X-ray absorptiometry		FVC	forced vital capacity
DIC	disseminated intravascular coagulation		GBM	glomerular basement membrane
DKA	diabetic ketoacidosis		GCS	Glasgow Coma Score
DMARDs	disease-modifying anti-rheumatoid drugs		GFR	glomerular filtration rate
DOT	directly observed therapy		GH	growth hormone
DRE	digital rectal examination		GHRH	GH-releasing hormone
DSA	digital subtraction angiography		GI	gastrointestinal
dsDNA	double-stranded DNA		GTN	glyceryl trinitrate
DVLA	Driver and Vehicle Licensing Agency		HAS	human albumin solution
DVT	deep venous (or vein) thrombosis		Hb	haemoglobin
EAA	extrinsic allergic alveolitis		HbA1c	glycated haemoglobin
ECG	electrocardiogram		HBGM	home blood glucose monitoring
ENA	extractable nuclear antigen		HDL	high-density lipoprotein
ENT	ear, nose and throat		HIV	human immunodeficiency virus
ERCP	endoscopic retrograde cholangiopancreatography		HLA	human leukocyte antigen
ESR	erythrocyte sedimentation rate		HNPCC	hereditary non-polyposis colorectal cancer
ESRF	end-stage renal failure		HONK	hyperosmolar, non-ketotic pre-coma or coma
ET	endotracheal		HPLC	high-performance liquid chromatography
FBC	full blood count		HPOA	hypertrophic pulmonary osteoarthropathy
FEV$_1$	forced expiratory volume in 1 second		HR	heart rate

HRCT	high-resolution computed tomography	**MRI**	magnetic resonance imaging
IBD	inflammatory bowel disease	**MRSA**	methicillin-resistant *Staphylococcus aureus*
IBS	irritable bowel syndrome	**MST**	morphine sulphate tablets
IC	intermittent claudication	**MSU**	midstream specimen of urine
ICU	intensive care unit	**MV**	mitral valve
IFG	impaired fasting glycaemia	**NASH**	non-alcoholic steatohepatitis
Ig	immunoglobulin	**NYHA**	New York Heart Association
IGF-I	insulin-like growth factor I	**NSAIDs**	non-steroidal anti-inflammatory drugs
IGT	impaired glucose tolerance		
IHD	ischaemic heart disease	**OGTT**	oral glucose tolerance test
INR	international normalized ratio	**PCK**	polycystic kidney disease
ITU	intensive therapy unit	**PE**	pulmonary embolus
LV	left ventricular	**PEF**	peak expiratory flow
LVH	left ventricular hypertrophy	**PEFR**	peak expiratory flow rate
JVP	jugular venous pressure	**PPI**	proton pump inhibitor
LBBB	left bundle-branch block	**PR**	pulmonary regurgitation
LFTs	liver function tests	**PS**	pulmonary stenosis
LH	luteinizing hormone	**PSA**	prostate-specific antigen
LMW	low molecular weight	**PTE**	pulmonary thromboembolism
MAOI	monoamine oxidase inhibitor	**PTH**	parathyroid hormone
MDR	multidrug-resistant	**PTP**	pre-test probability
MEN-1	multiple endocrine neoplasia type 1	**PV**	plasma viscosity
		PVD	peripheral vascular disease
MI	myocardial infarction	**QCT**	qualitative computed tomography
MMSE	Mini-Mental State Examination		
		RAS	renal arterial stenosis
MR	mitral regurgitation	**RAST**	radioallergosorbent test
MRA	magnetic resonance angiography	**RBBB**	right bundle-branch block
		RBC	red blood cell
MRCP	magnetic resonance cholangiopancreatography	**RF**	rheumatoid factor

RRT	renal replacement therapy		**TSH**	thyroid-stimulating hormone
rtPA	recombinant tissue plasminogen activator		**TEDS**	thromboembolic deterrent stockings
RV	right ventricular		**TTP**	thrombotic thrombocytopenic purpura
RVH	right ventricular hypertrophy		**TURP**	transurethral resection of the prostate
SBO	small bowel obstruction			
SBP	spontaneous bacterial peritonitis		**U&Es**	urea and electrolytes
SIADH	syndrome of inappropriate antidiuretic hormone secretion		**UKPDS**	UK Prospective Diabetes Study
SLE	systemic lupus erythematosus		**UMN**	upper motor neuron
SU	sulphonylurea		**UTI**	urinary tract infection
SVT	supraventricular fibrillation		**VA**	visual acuity
T₄	thyroxine		**VF**	ventricular fibrillation
TB	tuberculosis		**VSD**	ventricular septal defect
TC	total cholesterol		**VT**	ventricular tachycardia
TIA	transient ischaemic attack		**WBC**	white blood cell
TNF	tumour necrosis factor		**WCC**	white blood cell count
TR	tricuspid regurgitation		**WHO**	World Health Organization
TRUS	transrectal ultrasonography			

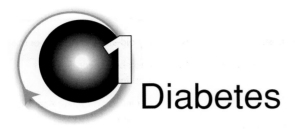

Diabetes

Steve Bain

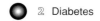

DIAGNOSIS

? **Questions for each of the clinical case scenarios given**

Q1: What specific questions would you ask the patient?
Q2: What investigations would you request to confirm a diagnosis?
Q3: What examination would you perform?
Q4: What would be the initial management?
Q5: What are the long-term sequelae?
Q6: What issues need to be addressed apart from blood glucose control?

Clinical cases

● **CASE 1.1 – A 73-year-old man with glycosuria and a finger-prick glucose of 11.4 mmol/L.**

A 73-year-old man is found to have glycosuria on urine testing as part of a new patient assessment. A random finger-prick test by the practice nurse using a modern, calibrated, glucose meter gives a level of 11.4 mmol/L. Arrangements are made for a repeat blood test after an overnight fast; this plasma glucose level is analysed by the local hospital clinical chemistry department and is reported at 6.7 mmol/L.

● **CASE 1.2 – A 57-year-old woman with lethargy and thrush and a fasting plasma glucose of 8.2 mmol/L.**

A 57-year-old woman presents to the surgery with lethargy. She has a long history of recurrent episodes of vaginal irritation, which had been formally diagnosed as candidal thrush on one occasion. Treatment with clotrimazole leads to a short amelioration of symptoms. A fasting plasma glucose level has been reported by the laboratory to be 8.2 mmol/L.

● **CASE 1.3 – A 21-year-old woman with a random finger-prick glucose of 18.9 mmol/L and urinary ketones.**

A 21-year-old woman who has always been fit and well visits you shortly after her honeymoon. She has been profoundly thirsty and noticing blurring of her vision. A finger-prick test in the surgery shows a blood glucose level of 18.9 mmol/L and a fresh urine specimen has both glycosuria and heavy ketones (+++)

🏃 OSCE Counselling Cases

OSCE COUNSELLING CASE 1.1 – 'Will I always have diabetes?'

A 53-year-old man is diagnosed with type 2 diabetes mellitus. He is treated with diet and subsequently oral agents. A couple of years after diagnosis, he begins to take his diet more seriously and takes up regular exercise. He loses weight and his glucose levels fall to such an extent that he is experiencing frequent hypoglycaemia. He is keen to reduce his medication and wants to know if the diabetes is disappearing.

OSCE COUNSELLING CASE 1.2 – 'Does having diabetes affect my driving licence?'

A 48-year-old man is admitted to hospital with newly diagnosed diabetes. He is discharged on twice-daily insulin and after 6 weeks has established reasonable diabetic control with no hypoglycaemia. He has previously driven heavy goods vehicles and is keen to return to work. He asks your advice about driving.

●— Key concepts

In order to work through the core clinical cases in this chapter, you will need to understand the following key concepts.

Diagnostic criteria for type 2 diabetes published by the World Health Organization and recommended by Diabetes UK (2000)

Diagnostic tests should use plasma glucose measurements, from a venous sample and performed in an accredited laboratory. Diagnosis should never be made on the basis of glycosuria or stick testing of a finger-prick blood glucose alone (although these may be useful for screening).

If symptoms are present (i.e. polyuria, polydipsia and unexplained weight loss), the diagnosis can be made on the basis of a single:

- random plasma glucose ≥ 11.1 mmol/L
- fasting plasma glucose ≥ 7.0 mmol/L

If symptoms are not present, two abnormal results (as above) on separate days are needed.

A fasting plasma glucose of 6.1–6.9 mmol/L is termed 'impaired fasting glycaemia' (IFG) and should be followed up by a formal glucose tolerance test to exclude diabetes.

'Impaired glucose tolerance' (IGT) is defined by a formal glucose tolerance test as a 2-hour plasma glucose of 7.8–11.0 mmol/L. This should lead to assessment of vascular risk factors and yearly screening of fasting plasma glucose.

Answers

 CASE 1.1 – A 73-year-old man with glycosuria and a finger-prick glucose of 11.4 mmol/L.

 Q1: What specific questions would you ask the patient?

A1

The detection of glycosuria has led to two tests to investigate the possibility of diabetes. The random glucose is elevated (≥ 11.1 mmol/L) but, as a single test, is diagnostic only when it satisfies two criteria: it must be a venous sample (not finger prick), analysed in an accredited laboratory, and it must be in association with symptoms of hyperglycaemia. So the patient should be quizzed about typical symptoms, which will include lethargy, weight changes (gain or loss is possible), polydipsia, polyuria, visual disturbance and infections (e.g. thrush, balanitis, boils). Even in the presence of symptoms, a diagnosis of diabetes cannot be made because this has not been confirmed by the fasting plasma glucose, which is < 7.0 mmol/L.

 Q2: What investigations would you request to confirm a diagnosis?

A2

This patient has IFG because his fasting plasma glucose is between 6.1 and 6.9 mmol/L. The guidelines suggest that IFG should be followed up by a formal oral glucose tolerance test (OGTT). This may confirm a diagnosis of: IFG, if the 2-h glucose is < 7.8 mmol/L; IGT, if the 2-h level is 7.8–11.0 mmol/L; or diabetes, if the 2-h glucose ≥ 11.1 mmol/L.

 Q3: What examination would you perform?

A3

Given the provisional diagnosis of IFG, there should be no evidence of diabetes-specific small vessel complications (retinopathy, neuropathy, nephropathy); however, large vessel complications are possible. The cardiovascular system should be examined for evidence of large vessel disease (carotid auscultation, palpation of peripheral pulses).

Q4: What would be the initial management?

A4

Assuming that diabetes is not subsequently diagnosed by an OGTT, the patient would receive general health-care advice about diet and exercise. Patients should be advised on an appropriate diet for treatment of diabetes (i.e. high carbohydrate, high fibre, low saturated fat, low refined carbohydrate) with weight reduction if appropriate. A target body mass index (BMI) of 25 kg/m^2 is generally quoted. Recommended levels of exercise are regular moderate physical activity for sedentary individuals and 30 min on 5 days a week for those who already take some moderate activity. Patients with IGT would be followed annually by means of a fasting plasma glucose level.

Q5: What are the long-term sequelae?

A5

Neither IFG nor IGT imparts any risk of specific small vessel complications and glycosuria related to a low renal threshold for glucose is a benign condition. However, a diagnosis of IGT increases the future risk of type 2 diabetes, and is associated with significant cardiovascular risk (in some studies, equivalent to the diagnosis of diabetes itself). It is assumed that IFG carries similar prognoses.

 Q6: What issues need to be addressed apart from blood glucose control?

A6

Cardiovascular risk factors need to be addressed, specifically smoking, lipid levels, blood pressure, exercise and obesity. Aspirin may be considered.

● **CASE 1.2 – A 57-year-old woman with lethargy and thrush and a fasting plasma glucose of 8.2 mmol/L.**

 Q1: What specific questions would you ask the patient?

A1

In this case, the presence of symptoms (lethargy, recurrent thrush) and the elevated fasting plasma glucose (≥ 7.0 mmol/L) are sufficient to make the diagnosis of diabetes which, given her age, is almost certain to be type 2. She should be questioned for other symptoms of hyperglycaemia (polyuria, polydipsia, visual disturbance, weight change) as well as symptoms relating to small vessel disease (tingling, burning of the feet) and large vessel disease (angina, claudication, etc.). A family history should be elicited and also a drug history to exclude the use of diabetogenic drugs (such as steroids and thiazide diuretics).

 Q2: What investigations would you request to confirm a diagnosis?

A2

The diagnosis is already confirmed and additional tests are not necessary. Most clinicians would request a measure of long-term glycaemic control (such as glycated haemoglobin [HbA1c]) as a baseline for future comparison.

Q3: What examination would you perform?

A3

The UKPDS (UK Prospective Diabetes Study) showed that 40 per cent of patients with type 2 diabetes have evidence of complications at diagnosis; examination should, therefore, focus on small and large vessel diabetic complications. For small vessel complications, this would involve examination of the ocular fundi through dilated pupils (or arrangement for this to be performed via a formal screening programme), and examination of the feet for evidence of peripheral neuropathy, in addition to their general condition and the presence of pulses. There should also be a thorough examination of the cardiovascular system. The patient should be weighed and a BMI calculated (weight (kg)/[height (m)]^2).

 Q4: What would be the initial management?

A4

Most patients with type 2 diabetes are given a period of non-pharmacological management. Dietary advice, preferably from a state-registered dietitian, should promote a diet high in complex carbohydrates but low in fat and refined sugars. If the patient is overweight (BMI > 27 kg/m^2) calorific reduction should also be advised. The benefits of regular exercise should be stressed where appropriate. The patient should be taught how to monitor the impact of these changes by testing either urine or blood (finger-prick testing).

These conservative measures are usually continued for at least 3 months unless the patient becomes more symptomatic, in which case oral medication should be started.

 Q5: What are the long-term sequelae?

A5

The patient is at risk of both small vessel and large vessel disease. Regular screening (at least yearly) should be performed for diabetic retinopathy, diabetic neuropathy and diabetic nephropathy. Blood pressure (BP) and lipids should be monitored and treated if necessary (below). All patients should be considered for aspirin prophylaxis.

 Q6: What issues need to be addressed apart from blood glucose control?

A6

Other cardiovascular risk factors include:

- Smoking: advise complete cessation.

- Lipid levels: in the UK, use of statins for primary prevention of coronary heart disease (CHD) should be initiated when the 10-year CHD risk is > 15 per cent. This figure can be calculated using the Framingham equation, which takes into account age, sex, BP, lipids and ECG changes of left ventricular hypertrophy (LVH).

- BP: treat initially with an angiotensin-converting enzyme (ACE) inhibitor or an angiotensin receptor blocker when > 140/80 mmHg.

CASE 1.3 – A 21-year-old woman with a random finger-prick glucose of 18.9 mmol/L and urinary ketones (+++).

 Q1: What specific questions would you ask the patient?

A1

In this case, the diagnosis is type 1 (insulin-dependent) diabetes until proved otherwise.

This is based on the presence of ketones in the urine. Answers to further questions will probably support this view but should not dissuade you from it. One might expect there to have been a short duration of symptoms (days to weeks), such as profound weight loss, polyuria, nocturia, lethargy and recurrent infection.

In the absence of ketonuria, especially in an obese Asian individual, there is the possibility of early onset type 2 diabetes, although this is by no means the 'epidemic' suggested by newspapers (and some medical journals). A strong family history of early onset type 2 diabetes (affecting siblings, parents and grandparents) may also point to one of the rare autosomal dominant forms of diabetes, but again ketonuria more or less excludes this.

 Q2: What investigations would you request to confirm a diagnosis?

A2

No laboratory confirmation is necessary.

Blood should be taken for a laboratory plasma glucose but this must not delay initial treatment. A baseline level of glycaemic control would usually be requested (HbA1c or glycated haemoglobin) and a screen for associated autoimmune disease (especially thyroid function) may be checked. Autoantibodies (e.g. islet cell, anti-insulin and antibodies to glutamate decarboxylase) are negative in 20–30 per cent of newly diagnosed cases and so are of little clinical use (they will also take some time to be reported). Insulin levels, likewise, are of little help and are not performed routinely.

 Q3: What examination would you perform?

A3

In a typical case of type 1 diabetes, there will be no evidence of diabetic complications at diagnosis because the duration of hyperglycaemia will have been short-lived. Assessment should focus on the conscious level and circulatory state of the patient because she could easily be acidotic, despite the relatively modest level of hyperglycaemia.

Q4: What would be the initial management?

A4

The patient needs to be treated with insulin and so should be in a setting where the necessary expertise is available (usually a hospital). If the patient is fit insulin can be started without the need for admission. Patients will need to be taught how to monitor blood glucose using finger-prick tests and to understand the concepts of hypo- and hyperglycaemia.

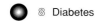

They will also need to be shown how to test urine for ketones and understand the significance of these. Dietary advice will be needed and appropriate targets for blood glucose levels agreed. Frequent contact over the early days and weeks after diagnosis will be essential, ideally with an experienced diabetes nurse specialist.

 Q5: What are the long-term sequelae?

A5

By virtue of her younger age at onset, this patient is at particular risk of the small vessel complications of diabetes, specifically diabetic retinopathy, diabetic neuropathy and diabetic nephropathy. The minority who go on to develop diabetic nephropathy (which usually manifests clinically after 15–25 years of disease) are prone to premature cardiovascular disease, as well as being more susceptible to the other small vessel complications.

 Q6: What issues need to be addressed apart from blood glucose control?

A6

The risk of specific diabetic complications and large vessel disease are issues that can be dealt with over the following months and years. Of a higher priority are matters that may have an immediate impact. The first of these is hypoglycaemia, which can occur from the moment that insulin injections are commenced. Patients need to be able to recognize the symptoms of 'hypos' and take appropriate action (see Case 1.15 and OSCE Counselling Case 1.10). They should also be aware that rapid lowering of blood glucose level can induce these symptoms, even when the blood glucose levels are within the 'normal' range. This patient should also be given counselling about future pregnancy. Exemplary diabetic control is necessary in the peri-conception period to reduce the risk of fetal abnormality.

👥 OSCE Counselling Cases – Answers

OSCE COUNSELLING CASE 1.1 – 'Will I always have diabetes?'

The answer is unfortunately 'yes'. This is certainly the case as far as medical and insurance matters are concerned. However, by strict adherence to diet and regular exercise, it may be possible to reduce, or even eliminate, the need for medication. This applies to both oral agents and insulin in patients with type 2 diabetes. In the case presented, medication should be decreased or withheld so as to reduce the risk of hypoglycaemia.

Glucose levels tend to rise with age, and so patients with type 2 diabetes who are on a diet will ultimately need oral medication (often labelled 'diet failures') and those on tablets may well need to go onto insulin.

People with type 1 diabetes may go through a period in the weeks to months after diagnosis where insulin can be withheld. This is labelled the 'honeymoon period' and is thought to reflect the removal of the influence of hyperglycaemia, which further depresses β-cell function. The continued (autoimmune) β-cell destruction ultimately means that insulin will be required.

The prospect for a cure of diabetes is some way off in type 2 diabetes, but may be possible for type 1. Recent advances in islet cell transplantation have allowed patients to become independent of insulin for more than 2 years. Unfortunately problems surrounding islet availability/preparation and tissue rejection mean that this remains a research procedure.

OSCE COUNSELLING CASE 1.2 – 'Does having diabetes affect my driving licence?'

The answer in this case is 'yes'. The Driver and Vehicle Licensing Agency (DVLA) issue regular guidance on the medical standards of fitness to drive. Licences are split into two groups (groups 1 and 2) with group 2 including heavy goods vehicles (HGVs) and buses (passenger-carrying vehicles or PCVs). This patient should be advised to notify the DVLA that he is taking insulin and that, while he does so, he is barred in law from driving HGVs. If the use of insulin is temporary he may reapply for a licence when he has been transferred to another treatment.

Regarding his group 1 (motor car and motor cycle) licence, he must notify the DVLA but he can retain his licence so long as he can recognize the warning symptoms of hypoglycaemia and is not experiencing disabling hypos. He should also advise his insurance company of his change in health status.

Note that regulations change and so readers are advised to avail themselves of the most recent DVLA guidance.

NOTES ABOUT GROUP 1 ENTITLEMENT (MOTOR CARS AND MOTOR CYCLES) IN THE UK

- Patients with type 2 diabetes managed on diet alone need not notify the DVLA unless they develop relevant complications (e.g. retinopathy affecting visual acuity or visual fields)

- Patients with type 2 diabetes treated with oral hypoglycaemic medication should notify the DVLA but will be allowed to retain their licence until the age of 70 years, unless complications cause disability (as above).

- Patients on insulin should notify the DVLA and must be able to recognize the warning symptoms of hypoglycaemia. There are the same provisos regarding visual complications. Licences are granted for 1-, 2- or 3-year periods.

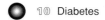

GLUCOSE CONTROL FOR PATIENTS WITH DIABETES MELLITUS

? Questions for each of the clinical case scenarios given

Q1: What are the treatment options?
Q2: What factors influence the choice of therapy?
Q3: What would be the preferred choice of treatment?
Q4: How would the impact of treatment be assessed?

Clinical cases

CASE 1.4 – A 72-year-old man with newly diagnosed type 2 diabetes.

A 72-year-old man has recently been diagnosed as having type 2 diabetes. He is mildly symptomatic with lethargy, thirst and polyuria. A random blood glucose level is 13 mmol/L and dipstick urine testing revealed +++ glucose but no ketones. He is a known hypertensive, taking bendrofluazide 5 mg once daily and his weight is stable at 94 kg (BMI 32 kg/m²). On examination, there is no evidence of large or small vessel complications.

CASE 1.5 – An 84-year-old woman with type 2 diabetes has been treated with gliclazide for 4 years.

A fit 84-year-old women with type 2 diabetes had been started on gliclazide after strict dietary adherence had failed to control her symptoms. She now presents with persistently high glucose levels (home blood glucose monitoring or HBGM 12–15 mmol/L) and has an elevated HbA1c level (9.0 per cent) despite taking gliclazide, 160 mg in the morning, 80 mg in the evening. She is symptomatic with lethargy, frequency and dysuria. Random fingerstick glucose is 15 mmol/L and urine dipstick shows ++++ glucose, ++ albumin and + haematuria. BP is normal, weight is 67 kg (BMI 24 kg/m²) and she has no evidence of retinopathy. There is early peripheral neuropathy and foot pulses are absent.

CASE 1.6 – A 57-year-old man treated with gliclazide 160 mg and metformin 500 mg three times daily, who has suboptimal glycaemic control.

A 57-year-old man with type 2 diabetes is currently treated with gliclazide 160 mg twice daily and metformin 500 mg three times daily, but his glycaemic control is suboptimal. He reports blood glucose levels between 12 and 20 mmol/L) and has an elevated HbA1c level (11.0 per cent). He claims good dietary adherence but is overweight (110 kg, BMI 33 kg/m²). He denies any symptoms and has previously refused to consider insulin. He has normal VA but fundal photography shows hard exudates encroaching on the left macula.

OSCE Counselling Cases

OSCE COUNSELLING CASE 1.3 – **'I have been diagnosed as having maturity-onset diabetes. Does this mean that I will never need go on to injections?'**

OSCE COUNSELLING CASE 1.4 – **'I hate doing injections and painful blood tests for my diabetes. Can I try an insulin pump instead?'**

 Key concepts

In order to work through the core clinical cases in this chapter, you will need to understand the following key concepts.

Glucose control for patients with diabetes mellitus

Type 2 diabetes is a condition caused by a combination of resistance to the action of circulating insulin (insulin resistance) and β-cell failure (lack of insulin). The loss of β-cell function is a progressive disorder, which is not modified by commonly used hypoglycaemic therapies (although more modern agents may have this benefit). This means that diet and then tablet therapies will ultimately fail and, if the patient lives for long enough, rising blood glucose levels will eventually require insulin therapy.

In the UK, the usual approach to glycaemic management is to start with modification of diet and exercise, often in the hope of achieving weight reduction (obesity is associated with insulin resistance). Unless the patient is very symptomatic or glucose levels are particularly high, this would be tried for at least 3 months. The target would be a HbA1c level < 7.5 per cent, although some would advocate lower levels (7 per cent). If the target is not achieved oral medication is added. Metformin is the commonly used agent, especially in obese individuals, because it does not promote weight gain and in monotherapy should not render patients hypoglycaemic. Unfortunately, it has significant side effects, including anorexia, nausea, abdominal discomfort, constipation and diarrhoea. These side effects are less pronounced if the dose is slowly increased, so 500 mg once daily is commonly prescribed, building up to the maximum of 1 g three times a day with meals, with weekly 500 mg dose increases.

If metformin is ineffective or not tolerated, sulphonylureas (SUs) are used. Gliclazide is the most commonly prescribed SU in the UK, starting at 80 mg once daily with breakfast and increasing to a maximum of 320 mg, usually in two divided doses. More modern preparations of this and other SUs allow for single daily dosing. As SUs act by increasing endogenous insulin secretion, they can promote both hypoglycaemia and weight gain as side effects.

In patients who do not tolerate metformin, or in whom SUs are ineffective, a glitazone may be initiated. These agents (currently rosiglitazone and pioglitazone are available in the UK) reduce insulin resistance and would, theoretically, be better used early in the treatment of type 2 diabetes. However, the guidelines of the National Institute for Health and Clinical Excellence (NICE) do not sanction this use; they are also contraindicated in combination with insulin. The use of all three classes of agents is now licensed in the UK.

There are various ways of starting insulin in type 2 diabetes: it can be added to oral therapy, usually as a single dose of long-acting insulin such as glargine or detemir, although the glitazone should always be stopped as a result of licensing issues. This regimen has the advantages of simplicity but is ultimately doomed to fail with patients needing fast-acting insulin to prevent post-prandial hyperglycaemia. This can either involve the addition of three pre-meal injections (a standard basal bolus regimen) or a change to two pre-meal injections of premixed insulin. As far as reaching HbA1c targets (6.5–7.5 per cent, the lower limit highlighting the risks of hypoglycaemia), the twice daily and add-on regimens are equally (in)effective and one can argue there is less activity going straight to twice daily insulin when tablets fail. This also has the advantage that patients can stop taking many tablets, although metformin is often continued to try to reduce the weight gain that can be associated with insulin use.

Answers

 CASE 1.4 – A 72-year-old man with newly diagnosed type 2 diabetes.

Q1: What are the treatment options?

A1

The treatment options are wide and include the following:

- Dietary review and manipulation
- Exercise
- Weight loss (achieved by diet and exercise although anti-obesity drugs may be considered)
- Change of antihypertensive agent
- Oral hypoglycaemic agents (metformin, an SU, acarbose, repaglinide, but not a thiazolidinedione or nateglinide because these are not licensed for monotherapy in the UK)
- Insulin.

Q2: What factors influence the choice of therapy?

A2

The choice of therapy is influenced by factors including the level of symptoms, the degree of hyperglycaemia, his weight and the fact that there has been no weight loss, and his age. This patient is said to have type 2 diabetes and this fits with his age, symptoms, obesity and hypertension. His symptoms are mild, glucose level is moderately elevated and there are no ketones in the urine. He currently takes a high-dose thiazide diuretic, which, in some cases, can cause glucose intolerance.

Q3: What would be the preferred choice of treatment?

A3

A reasonable course of action would be to advise on diet (see answer A4 to Case 1.1) with the aim of reducing daily calorie intake and increasing exercise. The bendrofluazide could be stopped and replaced with an ACE inhibitor. Assuming that he does not become more symptomatic, this regimen could be followed for 3 months at which point oral hypoglycaemic agents may be considered. The first-line agent would be metformin, based on his obesity.

Q4: How would the impact of treatment be assessed?

A4

The patient should be made aware of the symptoms of hyperglycaemia and make contact if these appear to worsen, especially if weight loss is marked. The technical options to assess the glycaemic response are near patient (usually self-) testing of urine or blood glucose and laboratory testing (HbA1c levels and fructosamine).

Home blood glucose monitoring is commonly taught to patients in this scenario, but critics argue that it is of little value and very expensive (in the UK more NHS budget is spent on monitoring than on oral hypoglycaemic drugs). Unless a patient or the clinician is going to manipulate therapy based only on the results of HBGM (and this is not the case here), one can argue that it should not be routine practice. The same could also be said of urine glucose testing.

Glycated haemoglobin and fructosamine levels provide a long-term indication of glycaemic control (HbA1c 2–3 months, fructosamine 2–3 weeks) and, if compared with a baseline value, will give a good indication as to whether conservative measures are being effective. HbA1c also allows for targets to be set, typically aiming for a level of 6.5–7.5 per cent (aligned with the Diabetes Control and Complications Trial [DCCT] assay).

Don't forget that a change in blood pressure therapy means that BP monitoring will need to be performed on a monthly basis and, if an ACE inhibitor is used, electrolytes will need to be checked beforehand and after 7–14 days of treatment.

 CASE 1.5 – An 84-year-old woman with type 2 diabetes has been treated with gliclazide for 4 years.

 Q1: What are the treatment options?

A1

The treatment options include:

- Further dietary review and manipulation
- Increase the dose of SU (gliclazide)
- Add another oral hypoglycaemic agent (metformin, acarbose, thiazolidinedione, repaglinide, nateglinide)
- Add or substitute insulin for gliclazide
- Exclude urinary tract infection (UTI) or treat if this is confirmed.

 Q2: What factors influence the choice of therapy?

A2

The choice of therapy is influenced by the natural history of her condition, her weight, her current therapy and her age. Type 2 diabetes is a progressive disease and so failure of diet and then oral monotherapy to control her symptoms should be anticipated (and not attributed to failure on the part of the patient). Although a dietary assessment is reasonable (and should be performed as part of the annual diabetes review), she has previously been strict and is not currently overweight. In this setting, it is unlikely that dietary change will make a significant impact. Her current dose of gliclazide is not the maximum recommended; however, the dose–response curve tends to be flattened at higher doses and so additional therapy would usually be instituted. Given her age, tight glycaemic control is not a priority and symptomatic relief with low risk of hypoglycaemia is the aim of treatment. Note that the possibility of diabetic foot complications does not influence the treatment choices

Although hyperglycaemia causes lethargy and frequency, dysuria with proteinuria and haematuria on dipstick testing suggest the possibility of a UTI (common in hyperglycaemia and a cause of worsened diabetic control). If confirmed by urine culture a course of antibiotics would be indicated.

 Q3: What would be the preferred choice of treatment?

A3

Add a second oral agent to her current dose of gliclazide. Thiazolidinediones are currently licensed for use in this combination only where metformin cannot be tolerated or is contraindicated. The use of repaglinide (an SU derivative) and nateglinide (an insulin secretagogue) with an SU is not recommended. Acarbose is poorly tolerated as a result of abdominal side effects (especially increased flatus) and so metformin would be the agent of choice. This should be started at a low dose (500 mg once daily for 1 week) and then increased weekly according to the blood glucose response, to a maximum of 3 g/day, so as to reduce the possibility of side effects.

 Q4: How would the impact of treatment be assessed?

A4

Given that the patient is already performing HBGM, it is not unreasonable for her to continue this practice and ask her to increase the dose of metformin according to the glucose response. Fasting, pre-meal and pre-bed glucose testing is the norm, with targets of < 10 mmol/L without hypoglycaemia being reasonable in this case. HbA1c testing could also be performed after 3 months for comparison with the pre-treatment level. The patient should monitor for side effects (which include any form of gastrointestinal disturbance) and reduce the metformin dose by 500 mg if these occur.

CASE 1.6 – A 57-year-old man treated with gliclazide 160 mg and metformin 500 mg three times daily, who has suboptimal glycaemic control.

 Q1: What are the treatment options?

A1

The treatment options include:

- Further dietary review and manipulation

- Increasing the dose of metformin

- Adding another oral hypoglycaemic agent (thiazolidinedione or acarbose)

- Replacing one of his current oral agents with another (repaglinide or nateglinide)

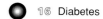

- Insulin
- Insulin and oral hypoglycaemic medication.

 Q2: What factors influence the choice of therapy?

A2

The choice of therapy is influenced by the natural history of the condition, his current therapy, age and weight, and the presence of retinopathy. The progressive nature of type 2 diabetes is such that all patients will end up on insulin if they survive for long enough. Although he is not on maximal doses of metformin, further increases are unlikely to achieve glycaemic targets. There is no evidence for greater efficacy of repaglinide or netaglinide over an SU in this setting, and the addition of acarbose is likely to have only a small effect. Addition of a glitazone (triple therapy) is an alternative but is often a disappointing combination in this type of scenario. So insulin becomes a leading option, especially given his young age and the development of diabetic retinopathy. Clearly the patient is not keen to go on to insulin and the reasons for this need to be explored, because many patients are pleasantly surprised at how painless insulin injections are (compared with HBGM). A dietary assessment is reasonable because weight gain on insulin is a real possibility and one may consider the combination of insulin with metformin.

 Q3: What would be the preferred choice of treatment?

A3

Suggest to the patient that he tries insulin for a period. This will allow him to see how simple the procedure can be and if, like many patients, he feels better on insulin he will wish to stay on it. Twice daily insulin using fixed mixtures before breakfast and evening meal is a simple regimen that may seem less daunting than basal bolus (where patients inject fast-acting insulin before each meal and a night-time injection of long-acting insulin). Given the risk of weight gain, he should continue on metformin but can cease taking his SU.

 Q4: How would the impact of treatment be assessed?

A4

Symptomatic improvement (he may recognize and admit to symptoms in retrospect, especially lethargy) and HBGM will provide feedback on progress. He should also monitor his weight.

ᴬᴬ OSCE Counselling Cases – Answers

OSCE COUNSELLING CASE 1.3 – 'I have been diagnosed as having maturity-onset diabetes. Does this mean that I will never need go on to injections?'

The short answer is 'no'.

Maturity-onset diabetes is the old term for non-insulin-dependent diabetes, now called type 2 diabetes mellitus. The natural history of this condition has been convincingly demonstrated and is one of progressive deterioration in blood glucose control. This is felt to reflect progressive loss of β-cell function over time. Insulin resistance, the other contributing metabolic abnormality, appears to deteriorate before the diagnosis of type 2 diabetes but then remains relatively fixed.

As a result of β-cell failure, dietary change is likely to have a limited and temporary impact, leading to the introduction of oral hypoglycaemic agents. Ultimately these agents will fail and the patient may need insulin to achieve reasonable glycaemic control. One can argue that, if an individual with type 2 diabetes lives for long enough, insulin is inevitable. This can be used as a justification for early exposure to the use of insulin (handling injection devices, experiencing the injection) so that, when insulin is needed, it is not delayed by unjustified fears.

The exception to this rule of progressive glycaemic deterioration may be patients who are obese at diagnosis and manage to lose vast amounts of weight, thereby restoring insulin sensitivity. There are also preliminary data that thiazolidinediones can slow the progression of β-cell dysfunction but these need to be confirmed.

LEARNING POINTS

- Type 2 diabetes is the modern name for maturity-onset (non-insulin-dependent) diabetes.

- The natural history of this condition is for blood glucose control to deteriorate over time, as a result of β-cell failure.

- If survival is prolonged, insulin treatment will be needed in most cases of type 2 diabetes.

- It is the treatment, not the patient, who has 'failed' and this should be expected and anticipated. Patients can be introduced to the concept of insulin at an early stage and should not be 'threatened' with its introduction.

OSCE COUNSELLING CASE 1.4 – 'I hate doing injections and painful blood tests for my diabetes. Can I try an insulin pump instead?'

Insulin pumps (also known as continuous subcutaneous insulin injections) are now available in the UK but this is not a good reason for using one because the amount of fingerstick testing is usually increased.

The use of an insulin pump involves the insertion of a cannula into the subcutaneous tissue, through which small amounts of insulin are continuously delivered. In addition, bolus doses can be administered by the same equipment, to coincide with meals. The pumps themselves are small devices (equivalent to a modern mobile phone) and can easily be carried in a belt/holster.

The NICE has recently (2003) advised that pump therapy can be made available to people with type 1 diabetes where multiple insulin dose therapy has failed to achieve good glycaemic control. Type 2 diabetes is not currently regarded as an indication for pump use. Patients should be able to maintain 'a high order of personal hygiene' (in order to avoid catheter site infection) and test fingerstick blood glucose four times a day. In addition, they should be capable of estimating carbohydrate and calorie consumption, programming the pump and changing the cannula site every 2–3 days. It is estimated that, in the UK, no more than 1 in 20 patients would satisfy these pre-conditions.

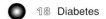

Although the NICE recommends that the NHS fund these devices, until now they have required self-financing and this has been an important issue. The devices cost about £1000 each and consumables amount to £700–1000 per year.

LEARNING POINTS

- Insulin pumps are available for therapy of type 1 diabetes in the UK.
- They are indicated where control remains poor despite multiple insulin injection regimens.
- Patients need to be highly motivated and technically competent.
- Cost may also be an issue.

DIABETIC SMALL VESSEL COMPLICATIONS

Q1: What questions would you ask the patient and why?
Q2: What investigations would you request?
Q3: What examination would you perform?
Q4: What are the differential diagnoses related to diabetes?

Clinical cases

⬤ CASE 1.7 – **A 75-year-old man with long-standing type 2 diabetes complains of difficulty in seeing the TV.**

A 75-year-old man with diabetes of 15 years' standing complains of difficulty in seeing the TV. There has been no pain or redness affecting his eyes and he has not had headaches. His diabetic control is poor but stable.

⬤ CASE 1.8 – **A 31-year-old man with type 1 diabetes has albuminuria on urine dipstick testing.**

A 31-year-old man with type 1 diabetes has joined your practice. He was diagnosed aged 12 years and, having attended the clinic regularly as a child, defaulted from the adult clinic, attending only when he needed replacement equipment (injection devices, etc.). He takes no other medication and has had no treatment for complications. BP: 160/80 mmHg; dipstick urine testing: +++ glucose, ++ albumin, + blood, but no ketones; visual acuity (VA): 6/6 in both eyes.

⬤ CASE 1.9 – **A 56-year-old man with newly diagnosed type 2 diabetes complains of pins and needles in his feet.**

A 56-year-old man is diagnosed as having type 2 diabetes by his local optometrist. He attends your practice and during diabetic review complains of 'pins and needles' affecting both his feet and his right hand. The symptoms are worse at night when he is in bed. Discomfort in his hand often disturbs his sleep. There is no discomfort in the feet during the day and exercise tolerance has been unaffected.

👥 OSCE Counselling Cases

OSCE COUNSELLING CASE 1.5 – **'Do all people with diabetes end up on kidney dialysis treatment?'**

OSCE COUNSELLING CASE 1.6 – **'My friend has diabetes and she says that all people with diabetes should go to a chiropodist. Is this true?'**

🔑 Key concepts

In order to work through the core clinical cases in this chapter, you will need to understand the following key concepts.

Long-term complications of diabetes are traditionally divided into diabetes-specific, small vessel complications (meaning that only patients with diabetes are at risk) and non-specific, large vessel complications (increased risk in diabetes but not limited to that condition). The small vessel complications are:

● Eye disease: diabetic retinopathy – the most common cause of blindness in the working population of the UK

● Nerve disease: diabetic neuropathy – usually a progressive peripheral neuropathy that presents with tingling and burning affecting the feet and progresses to complete sensory loss

● Kidney disease: diabetic nephropathy – the most common cause of end-stage renal failure in western economies

There is, however, crossover between the small and large vessel complications, e.g. patients with diabetic nephropathy have a greatly increased risk of ischaemic heart disease and most will succumb to this, rather than end-stage renal failure.

The diabetes annual review aims to detect diabetes complications at an early stage and institute therapy before there has been irreversible damage (e.g. laser treatment for retinopathy to prevent loss of visual acuity).

Answers

 CASE 1.7 – A 75-year-old man with long-standing type 2 diabetes complains of difficulty in seeing the TV.

 Q1: What questions would you ask the patient and why?

A1

Symptoms of cataract progression include halos around bright lights, such as car headlights. The symptoms are usually slow in progression but patients may report abrupt changes. Maculopathy may give either a slow or a sudden loss of vision in one eye whereas a bleed related to proliferative diabetic retinopathy classically causes sudden, painless, visual loss in one eye. Note that patients may be unaware of the extent of loss of vision if the good eye compensates. Changes in vision related to poor glycaemic control (usually enhanced long vision and difficulty reading) may affect both eyes and can be variable over short periods. During periods of poor glycaemic control (e.g. at diagnosis) patients should be advised against changing their lens prescription.

 Q2: What investigations would you request?

A2

In the vast majority of cases, the history and examination will be sufficient.

 Q3: What examination would you perform?

A3

Visual acuity should be tested, with correction (spectacles) if the patient normally uses these for distance vision. Pinhole correction should be performed if the VA is 6/9 or less. Examination of the fundi through dilated pupils (1 per cent tropicamide) is mandatory. This will allow detection of a cataract by examination of the red reflex and also detection of retinal abnormalities by direct visualization, including those concerning diabetes and related medical disorders. Ideally, binocular stereomicroscopy should be performed (usually in the setting of an ophthalmic clinic), which facilitates the detection of macular oedema. Digital images may also be requested.

A4

Q4: What are the differential diagnoses related to diabetes?

The major possibilities related to his diabetes are:

- Cataract
- Diabetic retinopathy (more likely maculopathy than proliferative diabetic retinopathy)
- Change in blood glucose levels leading to alteration in lens shape
- Related retinal disorders such as central retinal vein and/or artery occlusion.

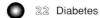

 CASE 1.8 – A 31-year-old man with type 1 diabetes has albuminuria on urine dipstick testing.

 Q1: What questions would you ask the patient and why?

A1

He should be asked about symptoms of UTI (frequency, dysuria, nocturia, haematuria, etc.) Although his attendance at clinic has been sporadic, he will have had urine testing previously, so he should be quizzed as to whether he had been told about urinary abnormalities (especially albuminuria) before. Previous blood pressure assessments would also be of value because this one-off reading may reflect anxiety-induced (white-coat) hypertension. A family history of hypertension and ischaemic heart disease are also more common in patients at risk of diabetic nephropathy.

 Q2: What investigations would you request?

A2

A midstream urine specimen (MSU) should be sent for culture to exclude a UTI. If excluded then formal assessment of the albumin excretion is needed; this can be by one of the following, depending on the expected compliance: 24-hour urine collection for albumin; timed overnight urine collection for albumin excretion rate; first voided urine for albumin:creatinine ratio (ACR). Blood should be sent for HbA1c to assess glycaemic control, lipids should be checked (total and high-density lipoprotein [HDL]-cholesterol) and creatinine. Haematuria is not typical of diabetic nephropathy and so renal ultrasonography should be arranged to exclude other causes of albuminuria (rare in this setting).

 Q3: What examination would you perform?

A3

People with type 1 diabetes and diabetic nephropathy are at high risk of other complications. The feet should be examined for evidence of peripheral neuropathy and reduced circulation. Coexisting diabetic retinopathy is almost inevitable and so arrangements for dilated fundoscopy should be made. Blood pressure should be repeated after a period of rest and then follow-up arrangements for more BP checks over the next 2–3 months to establish whether there is a persistent elevation. If diabetic nephropathy is confirmed a target systolic pressure of 125 mmHg is recommended.

Q4: What are the differential diagnoses related to diabetes?

A4

The major possibilities related to his diabetes are:

- UTI

- Diabetic nephropathy: the duration of disease (19 years) is typical and it is likely that his control has been poor (given the poor clinic attendance). In addition to the albuminuria, he has raised BP, which is part of the syndrome.

CASE 1.9 – A 56-year-old man with newly diagnosed type 2 diabetes complains of pins and needles in his feet.

 Q1: What questions would you ask the patient and why?

A1

Peripheral neuropathy symptoms (to which burning dysthesia may be added) are of gradual onset, typically worse at rest and in bed, when bedclothes can be particularly irritating. Autonomic neuropathy (rare) may also be present, with symptoms including gustatory sweating (facial sweating after meals) and postural hypotension.

Carpal tunnel syndrome (CTS) is common at night, patients often being awoken with discomfort and typically shaking the hand to relieve symptoms. Excessive use of the hands (e.g. painting) may also induce symptoms. It may be associated with loss (or change) of sensation in the hand and symptoms can be referred to the whole forearm. Once again, a gradual onset of symptoms would be expected and the other hand may also be affected.

Given the association of CTS with myxoedema, acromegaly, rheumatoid arthritis and osteoarthritis, symptoms of these conditions may be elicited.

 Q2: What investigations would you request?

A2

Nerve conduction studies will confirm a diagnosis of both peripheral diabetic neuropathy and CTS. They are most useful in the latter where surgical intervention can be considered when entrapment is confirmed. Bloods to exclude hypothyroidism should also be requested.

 Q3: What examination would you perform?

A3

Examination of the feet for abnormal sensation, using monofilaments and vibration sensation as screening tools. Ulceration (painless) should be excluded and skin care assessed. Peripheral pulses should be examined and may be 'bounding' in the neuropathic foot.

In CTS there may be sensory loss over the palmar aspects of the first three-and-a-half fingers and wasting of the thenar eminence. In advanced cases, there can be weakness of abduction, flexion and apposition of the thumb. Symptoms can be worsened by various manoeuvres such as percussion of the carpal tunnel (Tinel's sign), flexion of the wrist (Phalen's sign) and hyperextension of the wrist.

Given the association of CTS with myxoedema, acromegaly, rheumatoid arthritis and osteoarthritis, signs of these conditions may be looked for.

Q4: What are the differential diagnoses related to diabetes?

A4

The major possibilities related to his diabetes are:

- Peripheral diabetic neuropathy affecting the feet and possibly the right hand. Although recently diagnosed, the patient has clearly had diabetes for some time to manifest retinal changes. Hence, other long-term complications of diabetes may also be present.

- CTS affecting the right hand.

- A mononeuropathy affecting the right hand.

- Vascular insufficiency is an UNLIKELY cause of symptoms given the absence of claudication.

ÅÅ OSCE Counselling Cases – Answers

OSCE COUNSELLING CASE 1.5 – 'Do all people with diabetes end up on kidney dialysis treatment?'

No.

There may appear to be a paradox in that diabetes is now the most common cause of end-stage renal failure in the western world and renal dialysis as a result of diabetes is becoming more frequent. However, this relates to the massive increase in the numbers of people diagnosed as having diabetes, and the vast majority will never need dialysis treatment.

Taking the example of type 1 diabetes, studies from the 1960s and 1970s show that only a minority (at most 40 per cent) of patients will develop diabetic nephropathy, irrespective of their glycaemic control. This is likely to represent a genetic predisposition to diabetic nephropathy, which means that most patients are protected from this complication (contrast with diabetic retinopathy where all patients continue to be at risk). Continued improvements in BP, lipids and glucose control will inevitably reduce this proportion.

In type 2 diabetes, the major risk associated with abnormal albumin excretion is cardiovascular disease, which tends to cause premature death long before renal dialysis becomes a possibility. Although advances in the pharmacotherapy of BP and lipids may reduce the premature heart deaths, they are also likely to preserve renal function so that this largely elderly cohort will not end up on dialysis.

LEARNING POINTS

- Diabetes is the most common cause of end-stage renal disease in the western world.

- The number of people with diabetes going on to renal dialysis programmes is likely to increase as a result of the rise in prevalence of diabetes.

- Susceptibility to diabetic nephropathy is partly genetically determined with most patients protected from this complication

- With advances in BP, lipid and glucose management, the proportion of people with diabetes, especially type 1, needing renal replacement therapy is likely to fall.

- Diabetic nephropathy greatly increases the risk of other diabetic complications, including premature coronary heart disease (CHD).

OSCE COUNSELLING CASE 1.6 – 'My friend has diabetes and she says that all people with diabetes should go to a chiropodist. Is this true?'

No.

The level of resource directed towards diabetic foot care should be dictated by the individual needs. This has led to a risk categorization with varying levels of input.

NORMAL FEET (LOW RISK)

All newly diagnosed patients should receive basic foot health advice and subsequently be reviewed on an annual basis. This assessment can be carried out by a doctor, diabetes nurse specialist or practice nurse (with the appropriate level of training). If, at any stage, the patient is found to be 'at risk' or to have active foot disease, then referral should be made as follows:

AT RISK

Patients with reduced sensation, reduced pedal pulses or unable to perform nail chiropody (or have it provided by a responsible carer) should be seen 3- to 6-monthly for review by a chiropodist. Foot care advice should be given and the need for vascular assessment reviewed.

HIGH RISK

Patients with a risk factor for foot disease and either foot deformity or a previous ulcer should be seen 1- to 3-monthly by a senior podiatrist. Specialist foot care treatment and advice should be given, as per the published guidelines. There should be easy access to a shoe fitter, surgical appliances and, where necessary, a limb fitting centre.

ACTIVE FOOT DISEASE

Patients with active ulceration, cellulitis, osteomyelitis, a Charcot joint or foot discoloration should be seen urgently in a multidisciplinary diabetic foot clinic. In addition, any patient who has had an ulcer for more than 6 weeks should be referred for multidisciplinary assessment.

LEARNING POINTS

- All people with diabetes need foot assessment and advice at diagnosis and at least yearly thereafter.
- This can be performed by different health-care professionals, so long as they have been adequately trained.
- The intensity of clinical input depends on the risk categorization of each individual case.

DIABETIC LARGE VESSEL COMPLICATIONS

? Questions for each of the clinical case scenarios given

Q1: Are further assessments required before the italicized finding provokes a drug intervention?
Q2: If drug therapy were indicated, which would be the most appropriate choice of agent?
Q3: What sort of follow-up is indicated?
Q4: What other issues need to be addressed as regards cardiovascular risk?

Clinical cases

● CASE 1.10 – A 68-year-old man with type 2 diabetes and a *total cholesterol of 5.6 mmol/L.*

A 68-year-old man with type 2 diabetes has a new person check in primary care. He has no other significant medical history apart from diabetes and he does not smoke. His BMI is 32 kg/m^2 and he has no evidence of diabetic retinopathy or foot complications. BP 170/96 mmHg and urinalysis shows glycosuria ++ but no protein. A random total cholesterol (TC) is 5.6 mmol/L and triglycerides 2.3 mmol/L. He takes metformin 1 g twice daily and has an HbA1c level of 7.5 per cent (normal range < 5 per cent).

● CASE 1.11 – A 76-year-old woman with type 2 diabetes and a stable *blood pressure of 166/70 mmHg.*

A 76-year-old woman with type 2 diabetes is under regular review. She has a history of angina, which is well controlled, and does not smoke. Her BMI is 28 kg/m^2 and she has background diabetic retinopathy and absent foot pulses. BP 166/70 mmHg and urinalysis shows persistent + albuminuria in the absence of infection. BP recordings over the previous 6 months have shown similar levels. She takes gliclazide 80 mg twice daily, and isosorbide mononitrate 60 mg, simvastatin 10 mg and aspirin 75 mg once daily. A random TC is 4.8 mmol/L, triglycerides 2.3 mmol/L. and HbA1c 7.8 per cent (normal range < 5 per cent).

● CASE 1.12 – A 21-year-old woman with type 1 diabetes and *microalbuminuria* (urinary albumin:creatinine ratio of 2.7).

A 21-year-old woman with type 1 diabetes of 15 years' standing has an annual review of her diabetes. She injects insulin using a basal bolus regimen and does not smoke. Her BMI is 22 kg/m^2, BP 120/60 mmHg and she has good pedal pulses. She has minimal background diabetic retinopathy and slightly diminished sensation in her feet. Random TC is 5.7 mmol/L, triglycerides 1.1 mmol/L. and HbA1c 6.5 per cent (normal range < 5 per cent). Analysis of a random urine shows an ACR of 2.7 which is reported as 'microalbuminuria'. Previously urinalysis had been negative for dipstick proteinuria.

OSCE Counselling Cases

OSCE COUNSELLING CASE 1.7 – **'As someone with diabetes, should I be taking aspirin?'**

OSCE COUNSELLING CASE 1.8 – **'Why is my blood pressure so difficult to control?'**

Key concepts

In order to work through the core clinical cases in this chapter, you will need to understand the following key concepts.

People with diabetes get the same large vessel disease as those who don't have diabetes, but they get it earlier and it is more widespread

Cardiovascular disease: 75 per cent of people with type 2 diabetes will die as a result of ischaemic heart disease (IHD) and some studies suggest that IGT carries a similar cardiovascular prognosis to overt type 2 diabetes. This implies that glucose control is not the dominant issue, and is consistent with the limited impact of glycaemic control in the UKPDS. Contrast this with the major impact of blood pressure and lipid control.

Peripheral vascular disease: diabetes is the most common cause of non-traumatic lower limb amputation in the UK.

Cerebrovascular disease: stroke is two to four times more common in diabetic cohorts.

Hence there is a focus on CHD prevention (both primary and secondary) in diabetes management with attention to lipids, BP control (and to a lesser extent aspirin) and a sound evidence base. Microalbuminuria screening is also recommended in this context (as a marker of early vascular disease) but the rationale for this is less convincing.

Answers

 CASE 1.10 – **A 68-year-old man with type 2 diabetes and a *total cholesterol of 5.6 mmol/L*.**

 Q1: Are further assessments required before the italicized finding provokes a drug intervention?

A1

The total cholesterol (TC) warrants consideration in terms of primary prevention of cardiovascular disease. Issues are: whether fasting lipids are required, the potential impact of diet and what level of cholesterol justifies drug treatment. The guidelines are constantly changing in view of additional trial evidence.

Total cholesterol is not altered by recent food intake (unlike triglyerides) and so a fasting sample is not mandatory. Most clinicians would, however, repeat the lipids so as to include an HDL-cholesterol. This allows for the assessment of the patient's 10-year CHD risk using the Framingham or similar calculation. Framingham includes age, sex, diabetes status, smoking history, TC and HDL-cholesterol levels, and presence/absence of LVH on ECG. According to the Standing Medical Advisory Committee in the UK, a CHD risk > 30 per cent is a justification for the use of drugs for primary prevention, so long as the total cholesterol is > 5.0 mmol/L. (After results from the Heart Protection Study in 2002, the guidance about statin treatment may be changed. This placebo-controlled study showed that, in cases at high risk of CHD (including people with diabetes), use of statins produced benefit in patients with a TC > 3.5 mmol/L irrespective of their HDL-cholesterol. On these grounds, this patient would be treated with a statin, irrespective of other CHD risk factors.)

For most patients, diet has little impact on TC levels, and this is borne out by the large statin trials, which show a reduction of only 2–4 per cent in diet-treated patients.

 Q2: If drug therapy were indicated, which would be the most appropriate choice of agent?

A2

A statin, in a dose that provides a 25 per cent reduction in TC. In the case of simvastatin, 40 mg once daily taken in the evening should be prescribed and, for other statins, a dose equivalent to this (e.g. 20 mg atorvastatin). There is currently no evidence that fibrates or any of the older lipid-lowering drugs produce cardiovascular benefits in this case scenario.

 Q3: What sort of follow-up is indicated?

A3

Liver function tests (LFTs) and creatine kinase (CK) should be checked before initiation of statin treatment, but are probably not needed again unless the dose is increased. At the same time thyroid function tests could be requested, to exclude underlying hypothyroidism, which can raise cholesterol levels. Patients should be aware of the risk of muscle pains, which are rarely the result of myositis, and CK should be checked if they experience this symptom. Lipids should be repeated after 3 months of treatment and, if targets have been hit, checked on a yearly basis thereafter.

Q4: What other issues need to be addressed as regards cardiovascular risk?

A4

One needs to give consideration to glycaemic control, smoking, BMI, BP and drug therapy, although not in that order. The evidence that improving blood glucose control and reducing weight would have a major impact on CHD risk in this case is weak. In contrast, BP control is crucial; however, one needs to know that the reading taken on this visit is representative and not anxiety induced (so-called white coat hypertension). An ECG may be helpful, because evidence of LVH would imply long-standing hypertension; however, if this were normal then repeated BP checks should be arranged. A minimum of three recordings over a 3-month period would be appropriate with consideration of drug therapy if the level remains > 140/80 mmHg. Once again, additional dietary measures are unlikely to have much impact. Finally the patient should take aspirin 75 mg once daily unless there are known contraindications.

● **CASE 1.11 – A 76-year-old woman with type 2 diabetes and a stable *blood pressure of 166/70 mmHg*.**

 Q1: Are further assessments required before the italicized finding provokes a drug intervention?

A1

This patient with diabetes, IHD and peripheral vascular disease has isolated systolic hypertension confirmed by multiple assessments over time. The literature strongly supports reduction of her systolic pressure using drugs to a target of 140 mmHg. Further attention to weight, exercise and glycaemic control would be beneficial but they have minimal impact on her BP. Apart from baseline urea and electrolytes (U&Es), no further investigations are required at this point.

 Q2: If drug therapy were indicated, which would be the most appropriate choice of agent?

A2

The first-line antihypertensive agent in a person with diabetes and proteinuria should be an inhibitor of the renin–angiotensin system. Although this would usually involve the use of an ACE inhibitor, there is increasing evidence to support the use of angiotensin II receptor blockers (ARBs). Check that U&Es have been performed before initiation and 7–10 days thereafter. For a substantial proportion of people with diabetes monotherapy is not sufficient to achieve BP targets and additional classes of BP medication will be needed. A typical second-line agent in this case would be a low-dose diuretic.

 Q3: What sort of follow-up is indicated?

A3

The effect of drug therapy may take 2 months to become apparent. An interim target BP of 160 mmHg is appropriate and, if the patient feels well having achieved this, further increases in medication should be made aiming for systolic BP 140 mmHg. Once stabilized, BP can be checked at 3- to 6-month intervals. Patients on ACE inhibitors and ARBs should have renal function and electrolytes checked at regular intervals (about 6 monthly) because renal function can deteriorate at any time. Additional tests are required if the dose of ACE inhibitor/ARB is increased, additional medication is added or there is intercurrent illness.

 Q4: What other issues need to be addressed as regards cardiovascular risk?

A4

Attention to glycaemic control, weight and exercise is justified but unlikely to have a significant impact on CHD risk. One should review her other medications, increasing the simvastatin dose to 40 mg once daily (the dose on which most of the evidence for this agent is based) and increase the dose of aspirin which should be 150 mg once daily, given her known IHD.

 CASE 1.12 – A 21-year-old woman with type 1 diabetes and *microalbuminuria* (urinary albumin:creatinine ratio of 2.7).

 Q1: Are further assessments required before the italicized finding provokes a drug intervention?

A1

Screening for microalbuminuria in patients with type 1 diabetes is commonly part of the diabetes annual review. It aims to detect the easy stages of diabetic nephropathy, before the onset of dipstick-positive proteinuria (so-called macroalbuminuria). Diabetic nephropathy is a clinical syndrome of persistent proteinuria, hypertension and declining renal function. Patients with this complication have increased premature morbidity and mortality as a result of end-stage renal failure, cardiovascular disease and other diabetes complications, which cluster in this cohort. In well-controlled patients, the discovery of microalbuminuria after 15 years of diabetes would be typical of the natural history of this complication.

The issue surrounds the validity of this screening result. Urinary albumin excretion rates are highly variable, being affected by infection, posture and exercise, and this means that sampling procedures are very important. The test should be performed on a first-voided urine sample and, if positive, infection should be excluded by culture. If microalbuminuria is confirmed then a timed overnight collection should be arranged for assessment of the albumin excretion rate and, if this is also positive, a further two overnight collections should be organized. No treatment should be instituted on the basis of this one-off finding.

Q2: If drug therapy were indicated, which would be the most appropriate choice of agent?

A2

Evidence supports the use of ACE inhibitors to delay the progression of microalbuminuria towards diabetic nephropathy, even in the presence of normal BP. However, a further consideration in this case is that ACE inhibitors should not be used in pregnancy and so appropriate contraceptive measures should be instituted before prescription is considered.

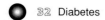

 Q3: What sort of follow-up is indicated?

A3

Once a definitive diagnosis has been made, annual screening is probably satisfactory. This is definitely the case if the repeat urine tests are negative. If a diagnosis of persistent microalbuminuria is made and the patient opted to take an ACE inhibitor, sequential urine testing is unlikely to alter management. Hence, yearly screening as part of the annual review would be appropriate.

 Q4: What other issues need to be addressed as regards cardiovascular risk?

A4

This person has no evidence of CHD and she is currently normotensive, non-smoking and lean. In this age group there is no evidence to support the use of long-term lipid-lowering therapy or aspirin, and she has good glycaemic control. Apart from advice on keeping her weight under control and taking regular exercise, no other issues need to be addressed.

👥 OSCE Counselling Cases – Answers

OSCE COUNSELLING CASE 1.7 – 'As someone with late-onset diabetes, should I be taking aspirin?'

'Late-onset diabetes' is an old term for 'non-insulin-dependent diabetes', now termed 'type 2 diabetes mellitus'. The short answer to the question is 'probably yes' unless there is a known contraindication to the use of aspirin. This advice, however, is based more on consensus expert opinion than on trial evidence.

Patients with known CHD should receive secondary prevention with aspirin prescribed at a dose of 150 mg once daily. For patients with no evidence of CHD, primary prevention with aspirin 75 mg once daily is slightly more controversial. The American Diabetes Association recommends that all people with diabetes who are aged 30 and over should receive treatment. In contrast, NICE guidance in the UK suggests that only those patients with > 15 per cent 10-year risk of a cardiovascular event should be prescribed aspirin and only when their BP is well controlled (systolic BP < 145 mmHg).

A useful compromise is to consider aspirin for primary prevention in all those individuals with diabetes who are prescribed a statin; this will be a significant and increasing majority.

OSCE COUNSELLING CASE 1.8 – 'Why is my blood pressure so difficult to control?'

Hypertension is commonly associated with type 2 diabetes, but is difficult to treat to target. This difficulty is made worse by the lowering of target levels, based on results of large clinical trials. In the UKPDS, BP targets were less stringent than those that are now advocated (typically 140/80 mmHg in type 2 diabetes); nevertheless, more than one-third of patients required three or more antihypertensive drugs. This difficulty is accentuated by the current consensus on hypertension management, which promotes the use of low/moderate doses of multiple classes of BP-lowering agents. The rationale for this is the epistatic interaction between drug classes (giving a bigger response than using maximal doses of a single agent) and the reduced incidence of adverse effects when drugs are used at lower doses. Added to this is the tendency for BP to rise with age and obesity.

All of the major classes of antihypertensive agents can be used in patients with diabetes and raised BP, and all classes produce an equivalent antihypertensive action and achieve target levels in a similar proportion of patients. Benefits of one class over another differ according to whether the patient has type 1 or type 2 diabetes, and whether the BP elevation is part of the syndrome of diabetic nephropathy. So ACE inhibitors may be preferred in patients with type 1 diabetes and microalbuminuria whereas ARBs may be first choice in patients with type 2 diabetes and proteinuria. However, results of the ALLHAT study imply that the cardiovascular outcomes are similar irrespective of which class of agent is used and the most important issue is the reduction of BP.

DIABETES EMERGENCIES

Q1: What is the likely diagnosis?
Q2: What investigations would be performed?
Q3: How would the diagnosis be confirmed?
Q4: What would be the initial management?
Q5: What are the potential complications?
Q6: What issues need to be addressed when the patient has fully recovered?

Clinical cases

● **CASE 1.13 –** **A 77-year-old man who is drowsy and dehydrated with a plasma glucose of 84 mmol/L.**

A 77-year-old man has been found collapsed at home by a care assistant. He was previously independent but known to have hypertension, angina and osteoarthritis. His regular medication was bendrofluazide 5 mg once daily, atenolol 50 mg once daily and aspirin. He had been noted to be lethargic over the previous few weeks and had been incontinent of urine on a couple of occasions. On arrival in the accident and emergency department (A&E) he was drowsy but orientated. Vital signs were normal but he was clinically dehydrated. Urinalysis showed ++++ glucose, ++ protein and + ketones. Plasma glucose was 84 mmol/L.

● **CASE 1.14 –** **A 32-year-old woman with abdominal pain and vomiting and a plasma glucose of 22 mmol/L and urinary ketones.**

A previously well 32-year-old woman presents to the GP surgery with a 24-hour history of abdominal pain and vomiting. On direct questioning, she admits to weight loss over the previous 2 weeks, associated with thirst, polydipsia and polyuria. A fingerstick glucose is 22 mmol/L and urine dipstick testing shows +++ ketones.

● **CASE 1.15 –** **A 18-year-old man, known to have type 1 diabetes, who is unconscious.**

An 18-year-old man who is known to have type 1 diabetes is found unconscious in his front garden. He had been playing football earlier in the day but had not complained of symptoms at that time. The diabetes was treated with four injections of insulin a day and his control was regarded as excellent.

OSCE Counselling Cases

OSCE COUNSELLING CASE 1.9 – 'What should I do with my insulin if I develop a vomiting illness that stops me eating?'

OSCE COUNSELLING CASE 1.10 – 'What advice do I give to my partner if they witness me having a "hypo" reaction?'

Key concepts

In order to work through the core clinical cases in this chapter, you will need to understand the following key concepts.

Hypoglycaemia

Hypoglycaemia in diabetes is caused by an imbalance of insulin (too much), exercise (too much) and glucose (too little). Patients usually experience warning symptoms and signs of hypoglycaemia, which prompt them to take treatment in the form of glucose. These are often listed as adrenergic (related to autonomic nervous system) and neuroglycopenic (brain hypoglycaemia); however, in reality patients will have warnings that are a combination of the two.

- Adrenergic: sweating, palpitations, hunger, tachycardia

- Neuroglycopenic: dizzy, faint, confused, abnormal behaviour, unconsciousness

Hyperglycaemia

Hyperglycaemia in type 1 diabetes may develop into diabetic ketoacidosis (DKA) and in type 2 diabetes hyperosmolar, non-ketotic pre-coma or coma (HONK).

Hyperglycaemic coma may be a presenting feature of diabetes or the result of intercurrent illness, manipulation of insulin (usually DKA) or concomitant medication (HONK). In many cases, the cause remains unknown.

Symptoms include lethargy, thirst, polydipsia, polyuria, nocturia, blurred vision and diminished conscious level although unconsciousness is uncommon (< 5 per cent). Patients with DKA hyperventilate (as a result of the acidosis) and have sweet-smelling ketones on their breath. They may also have mildly raised plasma glucose levels, so the severity of their condition should not be judged on this measure. Abdominal pain, masquerading as an acute abdomen, is frequently present.

In HONK, patients are severely dehydrated and glucose levels are always very high. The prognosis in HONK is poor as a result of the concomitant illnesses (CHD, renal disease, cardiovascular disease [CVD]) seen in this usually elderly cohort.

Answers

 CASE 1.13 – A 77-year-old man who is drowsy and dehydrated with a plasma glucose of 84 mmol/L.

 Q1: What is the likely diagnosis?

A1

Hyperosmolar, non-ketotic coma, which usually affects older people with type 2 diabetes and can be the presenting feature (as in this case). Precipitating causes include concurrent medication, including thaizide diuretics, and inter-current illness (a UTI being possible in this scenario). Although termed 'coma', it is unusual for patients to be unconscious. Although this patient has + ketones, this is unlikely to represent acidosis where > ++ urinary ketones would be expected. Extremely high plasma glucose levels may be seen.

 Q2: What investigations would be performed?

A2

- Venous blood for plasma glucose, U&Es, osmolality, bicarbonate, amylase and full blood count (FBC).

- Arterial blood gases (ABGs)

- Culture of urine and venous blood (and sputum if available)

- Chest radiograph

- ECG.

 Q3: How would the diagnosis be confirmed?

A3

Hyperglycaemia has already been demonstrated. Hyperosmolality can be confirmed after U&E results are available using the formula: $[2(Na^+ + K^+) + urea + glucose] > 350$ mmol/L. Plasma ketones should be within normal limits and there should be no acidosis confirmed by ABGs (or venous bicarbonate).

 Q4: What would be the initial management?

A4

- Attention to airways, breathing and circulation, as necessary

- Intravenous access and set up an intravenous infusion

- Cardiac monitor

- Treatment should then be given with intravenous insulin and intravenous fluids while monitoring electrolytes (Box 1.1)

- A nasogastric tube should be inserted and the patient should be fully anticoagulated with heparin

- Consideration should be given to central venous pressure (CVP) monitoring, urinary catheterization and broad-spectrum antibiotics.

Box 1.1   Hyperosmolar, non-ketotic coma (HONK)

Insulin management of HONK

- Insulin 3 units/h via intravenous pump
- Monitor glucose hourly using meter and laboratory testing
- Aim for fall in glucose level of 3–6 mmol/h
- At plasma glucose < 12 mmol/L, reduce to 1.5 units/h
- Continue insulin infusion for at least 24 h

Fluid management of HONK guided by central venous pressure line

- Intravenous 0.9 per cent saline if Na^+ < 160 mmol/L:

– 1 L in 1 h	Hour: 1	1 L
– 1 L in 2 h	Hour: 3	2 L
– 1 L in 2 h	Hour: 5	3 L
– 1 L in 4 h	Hour: 9	4 L

- Thereafter 4 hourly
- Change to 5 per cent dextrose when plasma glucose < 12 mmol/L

Electrolyte (K^+) management of HONK

- No K^+ in litre 1, pending laboratory reading:
  - **usually K^+ 3.5–5.5 mmol/L – ADD 20 mmol/L**
  - **recheck 2 and then 4 hourly**
  - if K^+ > 5.5 mmol/L – NO K^+ – recheck 1 h
  - if K^+ < 3.5 mmol/L – ADD 40 mmol/L – recheck 1 h
- **If Na^+ > 160 mmol/L, use half 0.9 per cent saline**

Q5: What are the potential complications?

A5

The prognosis for HONK remains poor (20–30 per cent). Patients are at high risk of thromboembolism and congestive cardiac failure as a result of the fluid regimen. As a result of age and co-morbidity, IHD, renal failure and stroke are common. Aspiration of gastric contents may occur in the setting of reduced consciousness.

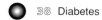

Q6: What issues need to be addressed when the patient has fully recovered?

A6

Despite the level of presenting glycaemia, management of the diabetes often does not involve insulin and some patients manage on diet only. The patient needs to be given dietary advice as well as specific diabetes education on issues such as monitoring, foot care, etc. This would usually involve the specialist diabetes nurse and a dietitian. Other aspects of cardiovascular risk need to be assessed and, in this case, BP medication may be changed from high-dose thiazide to an alternative class of agent (such as an ACE inhibitor).

CASE 1.14 – A 32-year-old woman with abdominal pain and vomiting and a plasma glucose of 22 mmol/L and urinary ketones.

Q1: What is the likely diagnosis?

A1

Diabetic ketoacidosis. This is an emergency complication of type 1 diabetes and can be the presenting feature, as in this scenario. Precipitating causes include intercurrent illness, e.g. UTI, and withholding insulin (in an established case). Abdominal pain and vomiting are not uncommon and can lead to the erroneous diagnosis of an acute abdomen.

Q2: What investigations would be performed?

A2

- Venous blood for plasma glucose (to confirm the fingerstick test), U&Es, osmolality, bicarbonate, amylase and FBC
- Plasma ketones may become a more widely used test with the arrival of near patient analyses
- ABGs
- Culture of urine and venous blood
- Chest radiograph
- ECG.

Q3: How would the diagnosis be confirmed?

A3

Confirmation of hyperglycaemia with ketonuria and acidosis (pH < 7.2, H^+ > 63 mmol/L). Note that the hyperglycaemia is often not pronounced and, indeed, may be absent.

Q4: What would be the initial management?

A4

The patient should be admitted to hospital. Intravenous access should be established for blood tests and infusion and a cardiac monitor attached. Treatment should then be given with intravenous insulin and intravenous fluids while monitoring electrolytes (Box 1.2).

Box 1.2   Diabetic ketoacidosis (DKA)

Insulin management of DKA

- Insulin: 6 units/h via intravenous pump
- Monitor glucose hourly using meter and laboratory testing
- Aim for fall in glucose level of 3–6 mmol/h
- At plasma glucose < 12 mmol/L, reduce to 2–3 units/h
- Continue insulin infusion for at least 24 h and no urinary ketones

Fluid management of DKA

- Intravenous 0.9 per cent saline:
  - – 1 L in 1 h   Hour: 1   1 L
  - – 1 L in 1 h   Hour: 2   2 L
  - – 1 L in 2 h   Hour: 4   3 L
  - –1 L in 2 h   Hour: 6   4 L
  - – 1 L in 4 h   Hour: 10   5 L
- Thereafter 4 hourly
- Change to 5 per cent dextrose when plasma glucose < 12 mmol/L

Electrolyte (K^+) management of DKA

- No K^+ in litre 1, pending laboratory reading:
  - – if K^+ > 5.5 mmol/L – NO K^+ – recheck 1 h
  - – if K^+ < 3.5 mmol/L – ADD 40 mmol/L – recheck 1 h
  - – if K^+ 3.5–5.5 mmol/L – ADD 20 mmol/L – recheck 2 and then 4 hourly

---

 Q5: What are the potential complications?

A5

The prognosis for DKA should be good, given that it affects young people who rarely have other significant co-morbidities. Cerebral oedema may occur during treatment, although the cause of this complication is unknown. Aspiration of gastric contents may occur in the setting of reduced consciousness.

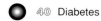

Q6: What issues need to be addressed when the patient has fully recovered?

A6

The diagnosis of DKA implies that the patient has type 1 diabetes and will require life-long insulin. She will therefore need to be educated about the condition, taught to inject insulin and how to self-monitor using fingerstick testing. She will need to be given information about the immediate complications of her condition (hypoglycaemia, DKA) and advised to avoid pregnancy until good glycaemic control is achieved. Ultimately she will need to understand the long-term risks of small and large vessel disease. These issues are best addressed by a diabetes nurse specialist and a formal education programme.

 CASE 1.15 – A 18-year-old man, known to have type 1 diabetes, who is unconscious.

 Q1: What is the likely diagnosis?

A1

Hypoglycaemia. As a general rule, an unconscious person with diabetes is hypoglycaemic until proved otherwise. This diagnosis is very likely in an otherwise fit young person who takes insulin. Precipitating factors in this case may be the exercise earlier in the day (the effects of exercise can last for many hours) and tight glycaemic control, which may provoke hypoglycaemia unawareness.

 Q2: What investigations would be performed?

Refer to Q3 answer.

 Q3: How would the diagnosis be confirmed?

A2, A3

Fingerstick blood glucose testing should confirm the diagnosis and is sufficient to allow initiation of treatment.

 Q4: What would be the initial management?

A4

In an unconscious patient the two main options are administration of glucagon or intravenous dextrose. Glucagon may be available because patients with type 1 diabetes are encouraged to keep a supply for this type of emergency. It comes as a powder that must dissolved in water (a vial of sterile water is part of the kit). One vial = 1 mg = 1 unit, which is the standard injection, usually into muscle (but it can be subcutaneous or intravenous).

Intravenous dextrose is given by diluting 50 per cent dextrose to half-strength and injecting 50 ml via a cannula. An infusion of 5 per cent dextrose is then set up to reduce the risk of phlebitis.

Q5: What are the potential complications?

A5

Patients can suffer injury if they have lost their warnings of hypoglycaemia. In older patients, hypoglycaemia may present with neurological signs typical of stroke. Death is thought to be uncommon in this setting, although hypoglycaemia has been implicated in the higher incidence of the 'dead-in-bed' syndrome seen in type 1 diabetes. With regard to the treatments, intravenous dextrose can cause phlebitis and glucagon is associated with nausea and vomiting.

 Q6: What issues need to be addressed when the patient has fully recovered?

A6

Need to find out the cause of the event (too much insulin, too much exercise or too little food) and then provide education in order to prevent future recurrence. In this case, the active issues would be manipulation of the treatment regimen to be able to cope with exercise and possibly a relaxing of glycaemic control in order to reduce the risk of hypoglycaemia and decrease hypoglycaemia unawareness.

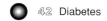

♟♟ OSCE Counselling Cases – Answers

OSCE COUNSELLING CASE 1.9 – 'What should I do with my insulin if I develop a vomiting illness that stops me eating?'

The issue here is what most people with diabetes refer to as 'sick day rules'. Patients will understandably be concerned that they may become hypoglycaemic by taking insulin without food. However, any intercurrent illness can cause blood glucose levels to rise, probably by increasing insulin resistance. Hence the advice that 'YOU SHOULD NEVER STOP INSULIN'.

Clearly they should perform more frequent fingerstick testing, at least 4 hourly. This will allow detection of hypoglycaemia and if, as is likely, glucose levels rise then additional insulin (rapid acting) may be needed.

For patients with type 1 diabetes, vomiting should raise the possibility of DKA and urine ketones should be checked at least twice daily. If these are positive to +++ or more then medical advice, and probably admission to hospital, must be sought. In young people with type 1 diabetes, dehydration can develop very quickly and a low threshold for seeking medical advice should be promoted.

Patients should be aware of the actions to take during illness and how to access appropriate advice (not NHS Direct). This will mean telephone numbers of the diabetes specialist nurse team and agreed guidelines for out-of-hours management of diabetes emergencies

OSCE COUNSELLING CASE 1.10 – 'What advice do I give to my partner if they witness me having a "hypo" reaction?'

Symptoms of hypoglycaemia include lack of concentration, bad temper, change in behaviour, confusion and pallor, all of which are easily (perhaps more easily) recognized by a third party. Hence it is vital that the partner of someone with diabetes be aware of the symptoms and signs of hypoglycaemia and able to take appropriate action.

If the partner suspects hypoglycaemia ideally he or she should encourage the person with diabetes to check a fingerstick glucose level. However, there is little to be lost by instituting treatment without confirmation of the diagnosis. Assuming the person with diabetes is alert this involves taking food by mouth, usually in the form of glucose tablets: 10 g glucose is equivalent to three sugar lumps or one Dextrosol tablet. Patients with diabetes should always carry some form of glucose replacement and Dextrosol tablets are recommended because they are less palatable than sweets (and so less likely to be consumed during normoglycaemic periods). Alternatives include 200 mL milk or 100 mL Coca-Cola (not Diet Coke). A longer-acting carbohydrate such as bread or biscuits should then be consumed.

If the patient is semi-conscious a glucose gel can be administered via the buccal membrane. Hypostop is a glucose gel supplied in a plastic bottle with a nozzle. The gel can be squeezed into the mouth between the teeth and cheek, and is absorbed into the circulation without the need for swallowing.

If the person with diabetes is unconscious he or she should be placed into the recovery position. If the partner has been trained, glucagon can be administered (see above), otherwise, medical aid should be summoned.

Perhaps the most important advice to the partner is not to panic and he or she should be reassured that the normal outcome of a 'hypo' is that blood glucose levels rise in response to the body's natural adrenergic response.

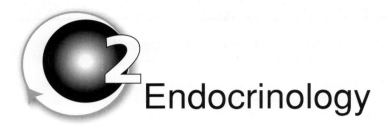

Endocrinology

Andrew Levy

HYPERTHYROIDISM

? Questions for the clinical case scenario given

Q1: What do you think the likely diagnosis is?
Q2: What tests could you do to confirm this?
Q3: What tests would help establish the cause?
Q4: What is the initial management?
Q5: What are the long-term complications/sequelae?

Clinical case

● **CASE 2.1 – A 26 year-old-receptionist presents with palpitations and weight loss.**

Although pleased about the latter, she is concerned that her menstrual periods have stopped and it is the anxiety related to this, she believes, that is responsible for disturbing her sleep. Her partner has insisted that she seek a medical opinion.

ÅÅ OSCE Counselling Cases

OSCE COUNSELLING CASE 2.1 – **'Do I have to have surgery?'**

OSCE COUNSELLING CASE 2.2 – **'Will I be able to have children after radioiodine treatment?'**

⚷ Key concepts

In order to work through the core clinical cases in this chapter, you will need to understand the following key concepts.

● Graves' disease is an autoimmune condition characterized by thyroid overactivity, eye changes (Graves' infiltrative ophthalmopathy or more specifically 'orbitopathy') and skin changes (pretibial myxoedema and finger clubbing, known as thyroid acropachy). The three components may occur in isolation, in any combination or never. Their clinical courses are usually independent and unpredictable. Skin changes are rare. Note that 'myxoedema' was an old term for thyroid underactivity. It is now a term reserved for the skin changes that sometimes occur in Graves' disease.

● In all hyperthyroid patients (even if iatrogenic), sympathetic overactivity leads to retraction of the upper lid with widening of the gap between the upper and lower lids when the eyes are open (the palpebral fissure). Increased exposure of the cornea and conjunctiva leads to grittiness and soreness of the eyes.

- In Graves' orbitopathy, which can occur without hyperthyroidism, autoimmune-mediated infiltration of the contents of the orbit and periorbital tissue leads to non-pitting and boggy soft tissue swelling, with increased volume of extraocular muscles, connective tissue and fat. This pushes the globe of the eye forward and can interfere with the function of the extraocular muscles, optic nerves and eyelids, reducing protection afforded by the tear film and leading to double vision and even blindness.

Hyperthyroid patients tend to be sweaty, tremulous, anxious and sometimes rather aggressive. Proximal myopathy (weakness of the thigh and arm muscles) makes their muscles ache and although tired, sleeping is often difficult. Appetite is increased, weight tends to decrease and stools are often softened but not frankly diarrhoeal. Fertility is reduced, and menstrual periods become lighter or stop altogether. Patients often find that their short-term memory is impaired, and it becomes difficult sometimes for them to make rational decisions.

In addition to sore eyes, the patient may complain of fast palpitations. If present, a thyroid bruit (the sound of blood rushing through the highly vascular, overactive gland) is a useful sign because it excludes thyroiditis and exogenous thyroid hormone as causes of hyperthyroidism.

Answers

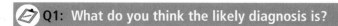 CASE 2.1 – **A 26-year-old receptionist presents with palpitations and weight loss.**

Q1: What do you think the likely diagnosis is?

A1

Hyperthyroidism would fit all of the symptoms here and, as it is very common, it is certainly an important diagnosis to confirm or refute. There are differential diagnoses of course, and panic attacks, agitated depression, tachyarrhythmias such as paroxysmal supraventricular tachycardia, atrial fibrillation or flutter, or excessive caffeine or other stimulant ingestion, could be responsible for some, if not all, of the symptoms. Of course, anyone taking thyroxine surreptitiously or being prescribed an excessive dose for treatment of hypothyroidism may also present in this way. Much rarer conditions such as phaeochromocytoma should also be kept in mind.

Q2: What tests could you do to confirm this?

A2

Laboratories vary in the thyroid function tests that they're willing to run for screening, but all would provide a measure of thyroid-stimulating hormone (TSH), which is suppressed by most causes of thyrotoxicosis. A free thyroxine (FT_4) is also useful, and will be raised above the upper limit of normal in hyperthyroidism. Unusually for tests of endocrine function, the TSH and fT_4 are very reliable and single samples taken at any time of day will be representative of thyroid function.

Q3: What tests would help establish the cause?

A3

Clinically, the presence of Graves' eye disease establishes the diagnosis in a patient presenting with thyrotoxicosis, and no further investigations need to be done. Similarly, if a thyroid bruit is present, this too is unequivocal evidence of primary hyperthyroidism, and excludes thyroiditis and the effects of exogenous thyroid hormones. Thyroid autoantibodies (antimicrosomal antibodies) are usually present, but this test is not often particularly helpful.

Imaging the thyroid either using ultrasonography or isotope scans is not often required in patients presenting with hyperthyroidism. Confirming the presence of a solitary 'hot nodule', however, can be useful because radioiodine is a more appropriate treatment than antithyroid medication, which although effective, would have to be continued in the long term to maintain euthyroidism.

Q4: What is the initial management?

A4

In this case, after suitable explanation of the various options, treatment with carbimazole at 40 mg daily, to which thyroxine (100 µg daily) is added after a couple of weeks is probably the most secure route to rapid restoration of euthyroidism. The patient must be warned that carbimazole can cause dangerous neutropenia idiosyncratically, and that the first sign of this is a sore throat. If this symptom occurs, the patient must be advised to stop the drug immediately and seek medical advice.

An alternative to the block and replace regimen described above is to treat with carbimazole alone and repeat thyroid function tests regularly, every 3–4 weeks, and to reduce the dose of carbimazole as the condition comes under control, aiming for a dose of 5–10 mg daily after 2–3 months.

 Q5: What are the long-term complications/sequelae?

A5

Abnormalities of thyroid function are very common and highly amenable to treatment. However, we often forget just how uncomfortable these conditions can be for the patient. Graves' eye disease, for example, can produce major cosmetic problems even if vision remains entirely unaffected. Primary hyperthyroidism often takes well over a year, if not longer, to treat effectively, and during this time the patient's ambient thyroid hormone levels, symptoms and mood often fluctuate uncomfortably.

Persistent hyperthyroidism is associated with osteoporosis, proximal myopathy and cardiomyopathy, manifesting as atrial fibrillation and its associated increase in thromboembolic risk.

👥 OSCE Counselling Cases – Answers

OSCE COUNSELLING CASE 2.1 – 'Do I have to have surgery?'

In the past, subtotal thyroidectomy was extensively used to treat hyperthyroidism. Radioiodine is a very effective treatment and antithyroid drugs are also safe to use in the long term if a patient objects to radioiodine, or if there is concern that radioiodine might worsen Graves' orbitopathy. Thyroid surgery is reserved for patients in whom very rapid and permanent control of hyperthyroidism is required, or in whom a goitre is causing compressive or cosmetic problems.

It is hoped that early and aggressive immunosuppressive treatment, principally with prednisolone, will reduce the frequency and extent of surgery required to correct problems associated with Graves' orbitopathy.

OSCE COUNSELLING CASE 2.2 – 'Will I be able to have children after radioiodine treatment?'

It is a commonly held misconception that radioiodine has an adverse effect on fertility, or that having children is inadvisable after radioiodine treatment. Neither is true. The only caveats to radioiodine use in this respect are that radioiodine has exactly the same effect on the thyroid of the developing fetus as it does on the mother. It is therefore vital that radioiodine is not inadvertently given to a woman who is pregnant. Health and safety regulations also seek to limit third-party exposure to irradiation and, for that reason, it is not an ideal treatment for anyone who cannot at least temporarily escape spending a great deal of time in close proximity to young children.

ADDISON'S DISEASE (AUTOIMMUNE ADRENAL FAILURE)

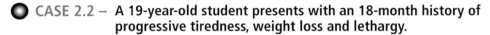

? Questions for the clinical case scenario given

Q1: What do you think the likely diagnosis is?
Q2: What tests could you do to confirm this?
Q3: What tests would help establish the cause?
Q4: What is the initial management?
Q5: What are the long-term complications/sequelae?

Clinical case

● CASE 2.2 – A 19-year-old student presents with an 18-month history of progressive tiredness, weight loss and lethargy.

One year before presentation she had a common cold that forced her to stay away from lectures for 2 days. Three months before presentation, another common cold laid her low for almost 2 weeks, during which time she lost 3 kg in weight. The local student health doctors had assured her that the symptoms were the result of either being pregnant or taking drugs. On examination, she was noted to have darker skin than her mother and pigmented palmar creases.

👫 OSCE Counselling Cases

OSCE COUNSELLING CASE 2.3 – 'Why did this happen to me?'

OSCE COUNSELLING CASE 2.4 – 'How will it affect my life?'

●— Key concepts

In order to work through the core clinical cases in this chapter, you will need to understand the following key concepts.

Before steroids (glucocorticoids) became available, autoimmune destruction of both adrenal glands invariably led to death from circulatory collapse. In much the same way that the autoimmune destruction of pancreatic islets, which characterizes type 1 diabetes mellitus, does not become apparent until many months after it starts, autoimmune destruction of the adrenal glands has usually been advancing for many months by the time it's recognized. In retrospect, the patient may have noticed progressive impairment of the ability to respond appropriately to stress, and that it is taking longer to recover from trivial illnesses such as the common cold.

Both adrenal glands, including the zona glomerulosa, the aldosterone-producing and the angiotensin II responsive layer, are entirely destroyed in primary adrenal failure. Consequently, the patient becomes critically deficient in both glucocorticoids (cortisol) and mineralocorticoids (aldosterone), resulting terminally in profound hyperkalaemia and hyponatraemia. Lack of glucocorticoid feedback at the level of the hypothalamus and pituitary leads to a marked increase in adrenocorticotrophic hormone (ACTH), which stimulates skin melanocytes. By making the patient look suntanned, the increase in skin pigmentation (including parts that are not exposed to the sun and new scars) tends to disguise the fact that the patient is gravely ill, and it can be surprisingly easy to overlook or ascribe the associated history of weakness, weight loss and intermittent vomiting to other causes.

In secondary adrenal failure (i.e. resulting from pituitary failure), lack of glucocorticoids is not as absolute, and catastrophic inability to respond to stress is rare. In addition, as ACTH levels are low rather than high, pigmentation does not occur and mineralocorticoid production is only modestly impaired because it is controlled by the renin–angiotensin–aldosterone pathway rather than the pituitary.

Answers

 CASE 2.2 – A 19-year-old student presents with an 18-month history of progressive tiredness, weight loss and lethargy.

 Q1: What do you think the likely diagnosis is?

A1

This is a fairly classic presentation of Addison's disease. It is relatively easy in retrospect to put the symptoms and signs of Addison's disease together, but it can be very difficult to recognize, particularly in its early stages, when adrenal function is only suboptimal under stress. Delay in diagnosis is therefore very understandable.

 Q2: What tests could you do to confirm this?

A2

The characteristic biochemical changes of hyperkalaemia and hyponatraemia tend to occur relatively late and, if the diagnosis is suspected, it is perfectly acceptable to start treatment with glucocorticoids immediately, pending an opportunity to carry out a diagnostic test. The confirmatory test (Synacthen) is described below under OSCE Counselling Case 2.3.

 Q3: What tests would help establish the cause?

A3

In the developed world at least 80 per cent of cases of Addison's disease are caused by autoimmune destruction of the adrenal glands. Tuberculosis (TB) remains a relatively common cause of Addison's disease in the absence of autoimmune disease, and is suggested by the presence of enlarged adrenal glands with necrotic areas and often dots of calcification visible on computed tomography (CT). In male children (aged < 16 years), X-linked adrenoleukodystrophy, diagnosed by measuring an increase in circulating very-long-chain fatty acids, is a common and important cause of adrenal failure. In older patients, measurement of anti-cardiolipin antibodies, a marker of primary anti-phospholipid syndrome, is useful if features such as recurrent venous thrombosis suggest that the condition is not idiopathic.

In primary adrenal failure, a random plasma ACTH will be high. In secondary adrenal failure, the symptoms and signs related to the condition are usually much more subtle and the biochemical signs do not appear. ACTH will be low or low normal and the cortisol response to exogenous ACTH will be suboptimal.

 Q4: What is the initial management?

A4

Glucocorticoid replacement (usually with 15 mg hydrocortisone first thing in the morning and another 5 mg at around 4pm) is required immediately and in primary Addison's disease, mineralocorticoid replacement with fludrocortisone

50–100 µg/day is also required. As Addison's disease is often disclosed by an episode of acute stress, it is not uncommon for glucocorticoid treatment to be given parenterally and at a higher dose at least initially.

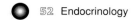 **Q5: What are the long-term complications/sequelae?**

A5

Patients with autoimmune Addison's disease are more likely to suffer other autoimmune diseases, and a proportion of them claim to 'not feel right' despite what appears to be adequate replacement therapy. Under conditions of stress, patients should be asked to step up their glucocorticoid dose by two- or threefold for a few days; they are asked to wear a MedicAlert bracelet or necklace and carry an injectable form of glucocorticoid with them to use if they find themselves unable to take oral steroids. For some patients, a longer-acting glucocorticoid such as prednisolone seems to be more comfortable than the short-acting hydrocortisone.

⚖ OSCE Counselling Cases – Answers

OSCE COUNSELLING CASE 2.3 – 'Why did this happen to me?'

All patients with autoimmune Addison's disease have detectable adrenal cortex and/or steroid 21-hydroxylase autoantibodies. The specific HLA (human leukocyte antigen) subtypes, HLA-A1, -B8 and -DR3 predispose to developing the condition. Having said that, it is not clear why some patients develop the condition and others do not. The risk of developing other autoimmune conditions such as type 1 diabetes mellitus, primary gonadal failure, hypoparathyroidism, Hashimoto's thyroiditis, vitiligo and pernicious anaemia is modestly increased in patients with Addison's disease.

If the diagnosis is suspected in an ill patient, formal diagnosis can wait and immediate treatment with glucocorticoids is usually appropriate. A high plasma ACTH in the presence of low random cortisol is often sufficient to confirm the diagnosis. If doubt remains, a cortisol response of less than 495 nmol/L 1 h after a 250 µg intravenous bolus of synthetic ACTH (Synacthen) confirms the diagnosis.

OSCE COUNSELLING CASE 2.4 – 'How will it affect my life?'

For most patients the diagnosis of Addison's disease has no adverse long-term effects on life or lifestyle. Some patients, however, claim not to feel as well as they did before the onset of overt disease, despite optimized glucocorticoid and mineralocorticoid replacement. For some of these patients, additional replacement of adrenal pre-androgens has been advocated, but there is little good evidence to support this at the present time.

The long-term outlook for Addison's disease is good, provided that the patient is fully aware of the implications of the condition and the need to respond to stressful situations by temporarily increasing the glucocorticoid dose.

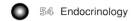

CUSHING'S DISEASE

? Questions for the clinical case scenario given

Q1: What do you think the likely diagnosis is?
Q2: What tests could you do to confirm this?
Q3: What tests would help establish the cause?
Q4: What is the initial management?
Q5: What are the long-term complications/sequelae?

Clinical case

● CASE 2.3 – A 56-year-old woman presents with depression, hirsutism, weight gain and muscle weakness.

On examination her GP found her to be hypertensive and to have wide, purple striae on her abdomen and thighs. Her visual fields were full to confrontation and there was no bruising.

ÅÅ OSCE Counselling Cases

OSCE COUNSELLING CASE 2.5 – 'Will "the tumour" spread to other parts of my body?'

OSCE COUNSELLING CASE 2.6 – 'Can I have tablets instead of an operation?'

●━ Key concepts

In order to work through the core clinical cases in this chapter, you will need to understand the following key concepts.

Hypercortisolaemia (Cushing's syndrome) is in most cases iatrogenic, an unavoidable side effect of the high-dose glucocorticoid treatment required for many immune and autoimmune conditions. Rarely, hypercortisolaemia is pituitary dependent (so-called 'Cushing's disease'), and is the result of a pituitary adenoma secreting ACTH. Cushing's syndrome can also result from other sources of ACTH such as carcinoid tumours of the lung or gut or from adrenal adenomas and carcinomas secreting inappropriate amounts of cortisol. It is often surprisingly difficult to identify the source of the problem with certainty and treat it adequately because even the most careful battery of well-organized investigations can be misleading. The first task is to confirm the presence of hypercortisolaemia and, if that can be confirmed, investigations are re-directed to identify the source.

In hypercortisolaemia of malignancy, there may be insufficient time for the typical phenotype to develop. In more chronic cases, patients characteristically gain weight, develop neuropsychiatric problems (often accentuation of pre-morbid personality – miserable people become more miserable and vice versa), proximal myopathy (difficulty standing from sitting without using the arms), muscle wasting, central accumulation of fat (filling in the temporal fossae and development of the characteristic 'moon face' and 'buffalo hump'), and weakening of the skin leading to the formation of wide, purple stretch marks (striae) and easy bruisability (although bruises are not often evident in the clinic). Hypertension, hirsutism (caused by increased ACTH drive to adrenal androgen production) and glucose intolerance are also common. In Cushing's disease the ACTH-induced increase in production of adrenal pre-androgens (responsible for the hirsutism) tends to protect against steroid-induced thinning of the skin.

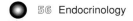

Answers

 CASE 2.3 – **A 56-year-old woman presents with depression, hirsutism, weight gain and muscle weakness.**

 Q1: **What do you think the likely diagnosis is?**

A1

Although Cushing's syndrome is suggested by the combination of mental and physical changes listed, the only one that is specific in the circumstances is the presence of wide, purple striae rather than pale striae. Simple, gross obesity could be responsible for everything else. Obese people are often depressed about their inability to lose weight, and the shear mass of tissue to carry around can make them feel weak, even though they tend to be much stronger than an equivalent patient with hypercortisolaemia. The fat tissue can aromatize pre-androgens to androgens as well as oestrogens, leading to hirsutism, and of course there is an association between obesity and hypertension, both of which are extremely common. Cushing's syndrome is an important diagnosis to make, but it is as well to remember that Cushing's disease is extremely rare, compared with simple obesity.

 Q2: **What tests could you do to confirm this?**

A2

If hypercortisolaemia is suspected, the best screening test available in the UK at the present time is the 24 h urinary free cortisol, three samples of which should be assayed along with creatinine clearance to ensure that the patient has managed to produce complete collections. Pregnancy, pain, heavy alcohol ingestion or alcohol withdrawal and vigorous exercise, particularly if the patient gets up very early every morning and runs, will increase urinary free cortisol to above the normal range. As cortisol is metabolized by the kidneys during filtration, if the patient drinks more than 5 L of fluid daily, urinary free cortisol will be high. In addition, some drugs unexpectedly increase urinary free cortisol (e.g. statins) or interfere with analytical methods, such as co-eluting with cortisol on high-performance liquid chromatography (HPLC) (e.g. carbamazepine).

Q3: **What tests would help establish the cause?**

A3

Establishing the cause of Cushing's syndrome can be difficult. Delays associated with various investigations can make it difficult to carry them out in a logical order without taking an excessive time to reach a conclusion. A peripheral ACTH measurement is useful because a very high level suggests ectopic ACTH syndrome and a very low level suggests adrenal disease. Pituitary magnetic resonance imaging (MRI) may show a macroadenoma (a tumour > 10 mm in diameter and/or distorting the sella turcica), in which case it is very likely to be responsible for the Cushing's syndrome. Conversely, as the prevalence of incidental pituitary adenomas < 4 mm in diameter in the general population is very high (probably around 10 per cent), finding one on MRI is insufficient evidence to send a neurosurgeon in after it. CT or MRI of the adrenal glands, showing a unilateral nodule with contralateral atrophy, suggests a primary adrenal lesion. For many patients, petrosal sinus sampling, i.e. sampling the venous outflow of the pituitary, is necessary to confirm or refute a pituitary source of excess

ACTH. The level of ACTH should be at least double the level found in peripheral samples taken simultaneously, and should increase further (to at least three times peripheral levels) in response to corticotrophin-releasing hormone.

 Q4: What is the initial management?

A4

The initial management of Cushing's disease (i.e. pituitary-dependent Cushing's syndrome) is trans-sphenoidal microadenomectomy by a skilled neurosurgeon. Obviously, if the problem is a carcinoid tumour of the lungs secreting ACTH, or an adrenocortical tumour producing too much cortisol, the respective tumours should be removed by an appropriate specialist.

 Q5: What are the long-term complications/sequelae?

A5

Unfortunately, cure of Cushing's disease is difficult to achieve and a large minority of patients relapse at some time or have only a partial remission and end up with persistent hypercortisolaemia. Improvements in trans-sphenoidal surgery and endoscopic adrenal surgery should allow a higher percentage of 'long-term remissions' in the future, and a reduction in the prevalence of patients suffering the consequences of persistent hypercortisolaemia, principally osteoporosis and the risks associated with impaired glucose tolerance or frank diabetes mellitus, hypertension and obesity.

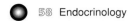 **OSCE Counselling Cases – Answers**

OSCE COUNSELLING CASE 2.5 – 'Will "the tumour" spread to other parts of my body?'

Metastatic spread of pituitary tumours has been documented but is extremely rare. The word 'benign' is, however, a little misleading in that some corticotrophic adenomas can infiltrate locally, particularly after bilateral adrenalectomy, which removes endogenous feedback inhibition of tumour growth (Nelson's syndrome). It is not unusual for corticotroph adenoma to be so small that, despite causing dramatic symptoms and signs, they are not visible on pituitary MRI. Even more curious is the relatively high remission rate when unaffected pituitary tissue is excised at surgery.

Cushing's disease has such a high risk of recurrence or failure of initial treatment that the word 'remission' is used rather than 'cure'.

Standard, fractionated linear accelerator (LINAC) pituitary radiotherapy to the remnant reduces recurrence rate about fivefold, but is associated with a small increased risk of other tumour formation in the radiation field and an increase in the risk of stroke. It is an important treatment, particularly if the patient has had bilateral adrenalectomy as part of the management of the condition.

Appropriate treatment of the primary disease does result in weight loss, but many patients find that it is difficult to shed all of the extra weight that they have accumulated before effective treatment was instigated.

OSCE COUNSELLING CASE 2.6 – 'Can I have tablets instead of an operation?'

Tablets tend not to be used first line because surgery offers the chance of immediate remission, confirmation of the diagnosis histologically, and an opportunity to debulk an adenoma that may subsequently be associated with 'space-occupying' problems if allowed to continue to grow *in situ*. Drugs are used sometimes in preparation for surgery or if patients have very aggressive disease causing severe neuropsychiatric symptoms, but they are often not very well tolerated. In the UK, metyrapone is used to inhibit adrenal hormone synthesis competitively. Ketoconazole, the imidazole antifungal agent, is also a useful adrenocortical hormone synthesis inhibitor, and etomidate, the imidazole anaesthesia-inducing agent, at very low dose is useful if rapid intravenous control of excessive glucocorticoid levels is required.

ACROMEGALY

 Questions for the clinical case scenario given

Q1: What do you think the likely diagnosis is?
Q2: What tests could you do to confirm this?
Q3: What tests would help establish the cause?
Q4: What is the initial management?
Q5: What are the long-term complications/sequelae?

Clinical case

 CASE 2.4 – **A 44-year-old woman presents with excessive sweating and an increase in hat size over a 3-year period.**

She comments that her face and hands just seem 'bigger' than before.

Key concepts

In order to work through the core clinical cases in this chapter, you will need to understand the following key concepts.

Acromegaly is caused by the presence of a growth hormone (GH)-secreting tumour of the anterior pituitary (somatotroph adenoma) that develops after puberty. Coarsening of the facial features, headaches, sweating and a progressive increase in jaw, glove, ring and shoe sizes are well-known features of excess GH. The most common and troublesome symptoms are, however, carpal tunnel syndrome, obstructive sleep apnoea and osteoarthritis, caused by persistent growth of soft tissue and cartilage. These changes can be partially reversed in some patients when the condition is treated, but, unfortunately, many of the changes remain and widespread arthritis, caused by disruption of joint cartilage, can be disabling.

If a somatotroph adenoma occurs before increased sex hormones cause the epiphyses of long bones to fuse at puberty, the patient has the potential to become a giant. In true gigantism, the somatotrophic adenoma not only arises early in life, but also impairs the function of pituitary gonadotrophs, giving rise to hypogonadotrophic hypogonadism. Without gonadotrophins (follicle-stimulating hormone [FSH] and luteinizing hormone [LH]), puberty cannot proceed and, if the epiphyses remain open, persistent growth of long bones can continue throughout life, leading in exceptional cases to remarkably tall stature.

As GH is primarily involved in the growth of the long bones, whereas sex hormones are responsible for growth of the axial skeleton, patients with gigantism tend to have very long limbs, but relatively small backs. These so-called 'eunuchoid' proportions, where each of the outstretched hands exceeds rather than equals standing height, are also found in other conditions associated with low sex hormone levels such as Klinefelter's syndrome (XXY).

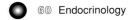

Obstructive sleep apnoea

Thickening of the tissues of the nasopharynx predisposes to severe snoring and frequent episodes of complete obstruction of the airways during the night. This leads to arterial blood oxygen desaturation and increasing respiratory efforts, causing partial wakefulness until eventually airflow resumes. Consequently, patients frequently complain of tiredness in the morning. Obstructive sleep apnoea has also been implicated in the pathogenesis of hypertension, which affects over one-third of people with acromegaly.

Treatment of acromegaly involves trans-sphenoidal debulking of the tumour and in some cases pituitary radiotherapy. Drug treatment is also used, with long-acting, parenteral somatostatin (GH-release inhibiting hormone) analogues such as octreotide LAR or lanreotide (Somatuline), dopamine (D_2) analogues such as cabergoline or bromocriptine, which reduce GH and insulin-like growth factor I (IGF-I) levels in about 10 per cent of patients, and GH-receptor blockers (pegvisomant). Surgery to relieve arthritis, nerve compression syndromes, snoring and facial deformity is also sometimes required. It is believed that acromegaly is associated with an increased incidence of bowel tumours, and patients in some centres are offered a routine colonoscopic screening when first diagnosed and at the age of 60 years.

Answers

 CASE 2.4 – **A 44-year-old woman presents with excessive sweating and an increase in hat size over a 3-year period.**

 Q1: What do you think the likely diagnosis is?

A1

Acromegaly is likely, of course. It should be remembered that there can be large discrepancies between circulating GH levels and the phenotypic changes that result. Some patients with very high levels of GH do not seem to develop many of the phenotypic features of acromegaly. Other patients with only modestly elevated GH levels sometimes continue to grow. Growth of the hands and feet is relatively pronounced because of the multiple cartilaginous interfaces between the many small bones. Growth of the skull is minimal and is a feature that is more characteristic of Paget's disease of bone. In acromegaly, increased hat size is the result of facial soft tissue growth rather than bony growth, although on radiograph and CT some skull thickening does occur.

Excessive sweating is also a feature of oestrogen withdrawal and thyrotoxicosis, both of which should be considered because they are much more prevalent problems, even though neither would explain the rest of this particular patient's symptoms.

 Q2: What tests could you do to confirm this?

A2

In many cases, the phenotypic changes of acromegaly are so obvious that little needs to be done to confirm the diagnosis. The condition might be 'burnt out', however, and, as persistent disease is an indication for surgery, it is important to measure a few random GH levels (three samples 20–30 min apart) and an IGF-I, as well as requesting an MR scan of the pituitary. The pulsatile nature of GH release means that a single measure of GH is not useful. If doubt remains about the diagnosis (and it doesn't usually), failure to suppress GH to < 2 mU/L after 75 g glucose orally confirms the diagnosis.

 Q3: What tests would help establish the cause?

A3

Rarely, acromegaly is part of the multiple endocrine neoplasia type 1 (MEN-1) syndrome, Carney complex or the isolated familial acromegaly syndrome. Somatotrophic adenomas have been described in association with GH-releasing hormone-secreting gangliocytomas in the region of the pituitary. However, the cause of acromegaly is ALWAYS a somatotrophic adenoma secreting too much GH.

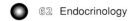 **Q4: What is the initial management?**

A4

In an elderly patient with co-morbidity, in whom somatotroph adenoma is unlikely to cause local, space-occupying problems, it is perfectly reasonable to do nothing. In a younger patient, trans-sphenoidal microadenomectomy or debulking of a macroadenoma is still first-line treatment. In terms of GH reduction, drug treatment with somatostatin analogues or the new GH-receptor blockers has a higher chance of success than surgery, but both are prohibitively expensive and, as far as we know at the moment, necessitate long-term treatment.

 Q5: What are the long-term complications/sequelae?

A5

Complications of acromegaly and its treatment are hypopituitarism, local space-occupying issues (such as visual field changes) and the effects of excessive GH levels on somatic growth and metabolism. Growth hormone is diabetogenic and acromegaly is associated with hypertension and an enhanced risk of cardiomyopathy (which might be specific to acromegaly), and respiratory complications related to altered chest shape and movements.

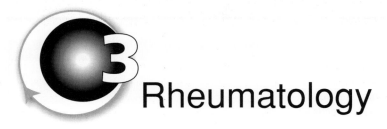

Rheumatology

Mark Pugh

POLYARTHRITIS

? **Questions for each of the clinical case scenarios given**

Q1: What is the likely differential diagnosis?
Q2: How would you investigate this case?
Q3: How would you confirm the likely diagnosis?
Q4: How would you initially manage the case?
Q5: What are the principles of long-term management?
Q6: What is the prognosis?

Clinical cases

● CASE 3.1 – A 38-year-old man develops painful and swollen hand joints.

A 38-year-old man presents with a 4-month history of pain and swelling of the knuckles, wrists, knees ankles and toes. He has no significant past history and the GP confirms the swelling of the joints and notes a history of more than 1 hour's stiffness of the joints in the morning. Initial blood tests reveal a microcytic anaemia of 11.8 g/dL and a C-reactive protein (CRP) of 9.6 g/dL.

● CASE 3.2 – Pain in the hands, knees and feet in a 46-year-old woman.

A recently postmenopausal woman presents with a 6-month history of pain and swelling in her hands, knees, neck and feet. The pain limits her ability to use her hands, and the knee and foot pain limit mobility. Apart from her joint pain she is otherwise well and there is no contributory past medical history. Examination demonstrates tender double bumps over the ends of her fingers, especially the index and middle finger, tenderness around the base of the thumb, limited neck movement, crunching knees with swelling and bilateral early bunions.

● CASE 3.3 – Knee pain in a schoolgirl.

A 16-year-old girl has a 6-year history of intermittent knee pain. She presented previously at the age of 10 also for knee pain, which was attributed to growing pains. Now she describes pain in the knees worse at the end of the day and especially bad after exercise. Her knees are often sore after sitting and difficult pain on ascending stairs has adversely affected school attendance. Knee swelling occurs sometimes. She also has pain in her hands, elbows and tops of her legs. Her joints often click so loudly that others pass remarks. She seems well in other respects and, apart from the previous assessment for knee pain, there is no past medical history. Her general practitioner detected no obvious joint problem and the full blood count (FBC), erythrocyte sedimentation rate (ESR) and rheumatoid factor (RF) were reported as normal.

👥 OSCE Counselling Case

OSCE COUNSELLING CASE 3.1 – **What can be done if I get a flare-up of my rheumatoid arthritis?**

🔑 Key concepts

In order to work through the core clinical cases in this chapter, you will need to understand the following key concepts.

Patients generally describe any pain around a joint as 'arthritis'. Arthritis, by definition, means inflammation of the joint and therefore in the absence of confirmatory signs should not be diagnosed. Arthralgia is the name for a painful joint without signs of inflammation. Pain can also be referred as well as originating from ligaments, tendons, muscles, nerves, arteries and skin around the joint.

There are a wide number of causes of arthritis which include:

- degenerative: osteoarthritis
- trauma
- infective: viral, septic, reactive, parasitic, fungal
- endocrine: hypothyroid, hyperthyroid, hyperparathyroid
- malignancy: paraneoplastic, secondary or primary malignancy
- allergic: erythema nodosum, drug induced
- autoimmune: connective tissue disease, seronegative arthritis, vasculitis
- crystal arthritis: gout and pseudogout
- congenital: Stickler's syndrome.

Answers

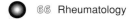

 CASE 3.1 – **A 38-year-old man develops painful and swollen hand joints.**

 Q1: What is the likely differential diagnosis?

A1

With a history of multiple, small joint swelling, more than 60 min of morning stiffness and a raised ESR, rheumatoid arthritis is a likely diagnosis. Other causes of arthritis need to be considered such as other connective tissue disorders, seronegative arthritis, infection, endocrine disorders, drugs and malignancy.

 Q2: How would you investigate this case?

A2

A full history and examination are important. Examination should confirm the presence of inflammation of the joints characterized by pain and swelling. All the joints should be examined as well as other systems, looking for evidence of systemic involvement and, of course, other possible causes of the arthritis apart from rheumatoid arthritis.

 Q3: How would you confirm the likely diagnosis?

A3

The diagnosis is clinical, with the presence of inflammation in the characteristic joints being sufficient to indicate it. The American College of Rheumatology Diagnostic criteria are often quoted, but the inclusion of erosions and rheumatoid nodules means that these criteria have low sensitivity in early disease. The presence of a high CRP and/or a positive RF are not always present in early disease, but if present suggest a likelihood of progression to early erosions.

 Q4: How would you initially manage the case?

A4

The initial management should be clinically to confirm the diagnosis and then perform baseline investigations including FBC, CRP (or similar measurement of inflammation), urea and electrolytes (U&Es), liver function tests (LFTs), and screen for RF and antinuclear factors. These tests should be consistent with rheumatoid arthritis and should not suggest an alternative diagnosis. The tests are also useful because many of the drugs used to treat rheumatoid arthritis are toxic. Radiographs of the hands and feet, and any other involved joints and chest, will often not demonstrate change but will be useful to monitor disease progression. The use of analgesics and anti-inflammatory drugs may provide some symptom relief while baseline investigations are undertaken. When confirmed rheumatoid arthritis patients should be offered disease-modifying anti-rheumatoid drugs (DMARDs) such as methotrexate, without delay to prevent the development of joint damage.

Q5: What are the principles of long-term management?

A5

The ongoing management of rheumatoid arthritis involves ensuring complete control of inflammation, monitoring joint damage, checking for other systemic manifestations and screening for the development of treatment side effects. As with the development of any chronic illness, patient education about the illness and its treatment is important to allay fears and promote treatment compliance.

Q6: What is the prognosis?

A6

Extra-articular manifestations of rheumatoid arthritis include:

- skin: ulcers and nodules

- lung: fibrosis, effusions and nodules

- neurological: myopathies and neuropathies

- eye: secondary Sjögren's syndrome and inflammation

- systemic: anaemia, weight loss and fevers

- skeletal: osteoporosis,

- cardiovascular: high incidence of cardiovascular disease and rare muscle, valve or pericardial involvement.

The progress for joint damage is: 5–10 per cent of patients do not develop damage; the rest do with 40–70 per cent after a chronic disease course and developing significant levels of damage and disability, and 20–40 per cent after a relapsing and remitting course associated with lesser levels of damage.

CASE 3.2 – **Pain in the hands, knees and feet in a 46-year-old woman.**

 Q1: What is the likely differential diagnosis?

A1

There is a wide differential; however, the presence of Heberden's nodes in the hands, a characteristic pattern of joint involvement and the absence of synovitis point to a diagnosis of osteoarthritis.

Q2: How would you investigate this case?

A2

Blood tests are not essential, but will help rule out alternative diagnoses. Radiographs of the symptomatic joints may demonstrate the typical changes of joint space narrowing, subchondral sclerosis, bone cysts and osteophytes.

Q3: How would you confirm the likely diagnosis?

A3

A history and examination should be sufficient to rule out alternative diagnoses and confirm the diagnosis. A radiograph is probably the most useful diagnostic test, but early changes can be subtle and it is possible to have osteoarthritis co-existing with gout or an inflammatory arthritis.

 Q4: How would you initially manage the case?

A4

Conservative measures should be addressed, including weight control, the use of padded footwear, e.g. trainers, and regular exercise. A walking stick can help knee symptoms and orthoses will help foot symptoms. Physiotherapy can alleviate local symptoms. Topical non-steroidal anti-inflammatory drugs (NSAIDs) or capsaicin cream provides some relief. Intra-articular steroids are safer than NSAIDs and may be appropriate to relieve joint symptoms. Analgesics are safer than NSAIDs and patients should always be encouraged to use paracetamol as a first-line drug. There is some evidence that complementary therapy may provide some symptom relief, with glucosamine probably having the best scientific basis.

 Q5: What are the principles of long-term management?

A5

The complications of osteoarthritis relate to the development of disability secondary to joint involvement. Patients can be reassured that, although activity may produce increased symptoms, only heavy manual work or professional level sports activity will accelerate joint damage. Treatment may produce complications, which may require treatment, of which NSAID-induced gastrointestinal damage is probably the most common. Surgery, especially of the knee and hip, is very successful for patients with significant pain and disability associated with significant radiological damage.

 Q6: What is the prognosis?

A6

Typically most patients are concerned about the development of future disability but can be reassured that this is very unlikely The key to successful management is to ensure that the patient self-manages the problem because cure is not possible and medical disease modification not achievable.

 CASE 3.3 – Knee pain in a schoolgirl.

Q1: What is the likely differential diagnosis?

A1

Benign hypermobility is the most likely diagnosis. An underlying inflammatory arthritis is unlikely as a result of the length of the history, the normal looking joints and the absence of inflammatory marker in the blood, but it needs to be ruled out.

Q2: How would you investigate this case?

A2

A history looking for pointers to alternative diagnoses, such as psoriasis, or systemic features of a connective tissue disorder or juvenile idiopathic arthritis, is important. A family history of joint pains in childhood is often present, highlighting a familial link in this disorder. Examination of the joints, looking for the absence of joint deformity or ongoing synovitis, would virtually rule out an underlying inflammatory arthritis. Radiographs and blood tests would be helpful to rule out alternative diagnoses.

✓ **Q3: How would you confirm the likely diagnosis?**

A3

Generalized benign hypermobility is diagnosed by demonstrating hypermobility in classic sites, including being able to bend the little finger to a right angle, bend the thumb back to touch the forearm, hyperextension of the elbow, and bending forward and placing the palms of the hands flat on the floor. Although normal on initial examination retropatellar pain can often be elicited by Clarke's test (compression of the patella with restricted knee extension). Flat feet are usually present. More unusual causes of hypermobility, such as Marfan's and Ehler–Danlos syndromes, should be considered.

 Q4: How would you initially manage the case?

A4

Reassurance that this is not the start of a deforming arthritis is usually very important. Anti-inflammatory and analgesic drugs offer some relief and can be important if the pain is severe enough to disrupt sleep or limit activities. Physiotherapy can improve pain by limiting joint movement through muscle development. Orthoses to correct flat feet and raise the heel can improve not only foot and ankle symptoms but also those from the knee, hip and back.

 Q5: What are the principles of long-term management?

A5

Occasionally these patients can have recurrent dislocations of the shoulder, hip or knee. This may require joint-stabilizing surgery but if possible should be avoided. On a day-to-day basis most of the problems relate to maintaining normal functions such as school attendance and physical activity.

Q6: What is the prognosis?

A6

Symptoms typically improve with age but improvement is not universal. Benign hypermobility does not appear to be associated with the development of early osteoarthritis.

‍🧍🧍 OSCE Counselling Case – Answer

OSCE COUNSELLING CASE 3.1 – 'What can be done if I get a flare-up of my rheumatoid arthritis?'

Patients can find the psychological impact of flare-ups difficult and need to be reassured that, even with a background of good control, flare-ups can occur. Sometimes no identifiable reason can be found to explain the flare-up; otherwise a waning of the effect of current medication, intercurrent infection or stress may be involved. Single joint flare-ups are usually easier to deal with than multiple joint problems. Patients should be advised to maximize their analgesic and anti-inflammatory medication, rest the affected joint and use ice packs. With no more intervention, the flare-up may settle. If it does not intra-articular steroid for a localized problem, or intramuscular, oral or intravenous steroid for a more generalized flare-up, may be necessary. A change in disease-modifying therapy may be indicated if the flare-up signals a loss of effect of the patient's current therapy.

MONOARTHRITIS

? Questions for each of the clinical case scenarios given

Q1: What is the likely differential diagnosis?
Q2: How would you investigate this case?
Q3: How would you confirm the likely diagnosis?
Q4: How would you initially manage the case?
Q5: What are the principles of long-term management?
Q6: What is the prognosis?

Clinical cases

● CASE 3.4 – An elderly man presents with a reddened, very painful and swollen ankle of short duration.

A 73-year-old man requires an urgent appointment for assessment of a painful left ankle. This started suddenly 2 days ago and is now so painful that he cannot put his foot to the floor. On examination the ankle is red and significantly swollen, but the rest of his joints are unremarkable. He has a history of two episodes of pain, redness and swelling of his right big toe, which settled over 2–3 weeks with NSAIDs and rest. Currently, he is on bendroflumethiazide for treatment of hypertension but is otherwise fit and well.

● CASE 3.5 – 'It all started when my second toe swelled like a red sausage.'

A 32-year-old woman describes a painful swelling of the second toe. This came on spontaneously 7 weeks ago. Examination of her other joints, including her back, reveals no abnormality of joint shape or function. While examining her joints you notice scaling patches of skin, with underlying erythema, over her elbows and knees. She has had these for 3–4 years and has treated it as dermatitis with simple cream. More recently she has noticed some flaking of her toenail on the end of the painful toe. The rest of the general physical examination is normal.

● CASE 3.6 – A 50-year-old man with a painful knee.

A 50-year-old travelling salesman presents with difficult pain in his right knee after he has been driving for more than 1 hour. This has been coming on for the last 3 years. He describes discomfort while walking up stairs and occasional pain in his knee in bed at night. Typically he has few symptoms earlier in the day but his knee aches by the end of the day. On review of his musculoskeletal system, he has a history of low back pain, and pain in the ends of his fingers, the base of the thumb and big toe. He had a cartilage operation on his right knee at the age of 29 after a football injury.

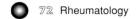

👥 OSCE Counselling Case

OSCE COUNSELLING CASE 3.2 – 'I am not keen on taking medication every day. Is there anything else I can do to help my osteoarthritis?'

🔑 Key concepts

In order to work through the core clinical cases in this chapter, you will need to understand the following key concepts.

Monoarthritis is usually caused by a different diagnosis to polyarthritis, although there is some overlap. Septic arthritis is typically monoarticular and therefore joint aspiration is a more important investigation in this group of patients than in patients with polyarthritis. Aspiration can both aid diagnosis and be of therapeutic value. Septic arthritis requires prolonged antibiotic treatment and every effort should be made to confirm the diagnosis before treatment is started. Most peripheral joints can be aspirated at the bedside; however, hip joint aspiration is usually best done with ultrasonic guidance. Other causes of monoarthritis include osteoarthritis, crystal arthritis (e.g. gout), sarcoidosis and seronegative arthritis.

Answers

 CASE 3.4 – An elderly man presents with a reddened, very painful and swollen ankle of short duration.

Q1: What is the likely differential diagnosis?

A1

With a similar history of self-limiting arthritis in the toe and a risk factor for hyperuricaemia with diuretic therapy, the most likely diagnosis is gout. The diagnosis not to miss is septic arthritis. This could also represent an alternative crystal arthropathy or an intermittent seronegative or rheumatoid arthritis.

Q2: How would you investigate this case?

A2

At the time of the attack there is typically a high ESR with raised white blood cell (WBC) and platelet count. The serum urate is sometimes decreased during an acute attack, producing a falsely normal-looking serum urate level. Hyperuricaemia is common in gout but not essential and a normal urate level does not exclude it. Factors associated with gout include alcohol, warfarin therapy, low-dose aspirin, myelproliferative disorders, tumour lysis, psoriasis and renal function. Tophi show up on radiographs and gout can produce a typical pattern of joint damage, although radiological findings are not always present.

Q3: How would you confirm the likely diagnosis?

A3

The definitive diagnostic test would be joint aspiration of the affected joint with the demonstration of urate crystals under a polarizing microscope; appropriate microbiological assessment should also rule out sepsis. Identification of urate crystals from another larger and possibly easier to aspirate joint, tophus or bursa would be virtually diagnostic.

Q4: How would you initially manage the case?

A4

The initial management of gout attempts to control pain and promote resolution of the acute attack. Rest is advised and patients should be well hydrated. If gout is secondary to an underlying medical problem such as renal failure this may need addressing. Provided that there are no contraindications, medical options include NSAIDs, colchicine, and intramuscular or intra-articular steroids. If nothing else, the attack should settle spontaneously in 4 weeks.

Q5: What are the principles of long-term management?

A5

Prophylactic treatment should not be started until 2–3 weeks after the acute event (due to the risk of exacerbation). Once recovered from the acute attack it may be necessary to start prophylactic treatment. The most commonly used drug is allopurinol, which is started in low dose and titrated upwards balanced against normalization of the hyperuricaemia. The drug is usually well tolerated but, in the event of problems such as rash and occasional leukopenia, alternatives include the uricosurics probenecid and sulfinpyrazone or low-dose daily colchicine.

 Q6: What is the prognosis?

A6

Repeated attacks of gout can damage the underlying joint. The associated hyperuricaemia may produce a nephropathy and/or renal stones. However, provided that the hyperuricaemia can be controlled by correcting the cause or using specific therapy, the outlook for this condition is very good.

● CASE 3.5 – 'It all started when my second toe swelled like a red sausage.'

 Q1: What is the likely differential diagnosis?

A1

The rash is likely to be psoriasis and the dactylitis is most probably associated psoriatic arthritis. Infection and gout can produce dactylitis.

 Q2: How would you investigate this case?

A2

Examination of the flexures and scalp may reveal additional psoriasis. Further examination of the fingernails may reveal characteristic nail pitting. A radiograph of the toe will most probably reveal little of diagnostic value but, as psoriatic arthritis is typically a chronic problem, one should be done for baseline assessment to allow future mapping of possible damage. Routine blood testing will usually reveal a raised inflammatory response.

 Q3: How would you confirm the likely diagnosis?

A3

The diagnosis is clinical based on a picture of a distal small joint and predominantly lower limb large joint arthritis in association with, or with a history of, psoriasis. Routine testing should not point to another diagnosis.

Q4: How would you initially manage the case?

A4

The first aim should be to control her pain. Anti-inflammatory medication may settle the attack; intra-articular steroid injection may also help. Some patients need to start taking DMARDs to control the problem. Anti-tumour necrosis factor (TNF) therapy can be used in patients with resistant disease.

 Q5: What are the principles of long-term management?

A5

This may represent the start of a chronic and possibly more widespread problem requiring long-term therapy. It should always be borne in mind that in the future she may develop associated ankylosing spondylitis, iritis, inflammatory bowel disease and genitourinary tract inflammation.

 Q6: What is the prognosis?

A6

The prognosis depends on the number of joints involved. Limited joint involvement has an excellent long-term outlook, whereas multiple joint involvement has a prognosis similar to chronic progressive rheumatoid arthritis.

 CASE 3.6 – A 50-year-old man with a painful knee.

 Q1: What is the likely differential diagnosis?

A1

Based on the history of previous cartilage surgery and pain on exercise at the end of the day, as well as pain in typical sites, osteoarthritis is the most likely diagnosis.

 Q2: How would you investigate this case?

A2

The most useful single investigation would be a weight-bearing radiograph of the knee. Radiographs of the other sites may also reveal degenerative changes. Blood tests looking for alternative diagnoses may be helpful.

Q3: How would you confirm the likely diagnosis?

A3

The absence of any other cause of arthritis and the presence of the typical radiological changes of osteoarthritis, including joint space narrowing, subchondral sclerosis, subchondral bone cysts and osteophytes, should be sufficient. Examination of the knee may demonstrate a joint effusion, decreased joint movement with discomfort and possible crepitus.

 Q4: How would you initially manage the case?

A4

Aspiration of the knee may ease symptoms, especially when combined with intra-articular steroid injection. Physiotherapy may be able to relieve symptoms. Simple analgesics and/or NSAIDs may provide additional relief.

Q5: What are the principles of long-term management?

A5

Osteoarthritis is not associated primarily with systemic complications but drug treatment is and therefore should be used judiciously.

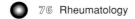 **Q6: What is the prognosis?**

A6

Full recovery is unlikely and the chronic nature of the problem may threaten this man's livelihood. Consideration should be given to advice about an automatic car or possibly a change in position in his company if his symptoms cannot be helped. Surgical treatment may be necessary in the longer term but is not inevitable.

👥 OSCE Counselling Case – Answer

OSCE COUNSELLING CASE 3.2 – 'I am not keen on taking medication every day. Is there anything else I can do to help my osteoarthritis?'

Patient concerns about medication can sometimes be allayed by discussion about the risks and benefits of medication. Education about the nature of the condition will promote independence. Reducing obesity, minimizing traumatic activity and using padded footwear will improve the prognosis. Orthoses can improve the symptoms of foot osteoarthritis and a walking stick can help mobility in patients with knee and hip osteoarthritis. Regular exercise aimed at improving aerobic fitness, muscle strength and proprioception will also improve mobility. Other forms of physiotherapy can be used to treat local symptoms. Many patients who dislike the idea of taking oral medication are happy to consider topical treatment in the form of NSAIDs or capsaicin. Intra-articular steroids or hyaluronic acid derivatives can also help symptoms. Patients often prefer to take complementary therapy and, in the case of osteoarthritis of the knee, glucosamine is proved to have modest symptom-relieving properties with safety, and controversially may also improve cartilage.

SYSTEMIC RHEUMATOLOGICAL ILLNESSES

? **Questions for each of the clinical case scenarios given**

Q1: What is the likely differential diagnosis?
Q2: How would you investigate this case?
Q3: How would you confirm the likely diagnosis?
Q4: How would you initially manage the case?
Q5: What are the principles of long-term management?
Q6: What is the prognosis?

Clinical cases

● CASE 3.7 – A young woman with joint pains and feeling unwell.

A 29-year-old woman presents with a 6-month history of pain and swelling, which started in the fingers and wrists and then spread to her shoulders, knees and ankles. She was treated for pleurisy twice 4 and 3 months ago and since then says she feels unwell. Most recently she says that she has developed a rash on her cheeks and forehead.

● CASE 3.8 – 'You've seen me before with sinusitis. Now I feel terrible, my eye is sore and I think I coughed up blood today.'

A 49-year-old man feels unwell with temperatures, myalgias, and pain in his wrists, knees and ankles. He is loosing weight and cannot work. His left eye has become increasingly sore and red. For some time he has had a cough productive of yellow/white sputum but today coughed up red blood. Investigations reveal a haemoglobin (Hb) of 10.8 g/dL, white cell count (WCC) of 14.8×10^9/L and ESR of 98 mm/h. Urinalysis demonstrated blood +++ and protein ++. Apart from a 3-year history of sinusitis requiring antibiotics and nasal spray, there is no significant past medical history.

● CASE 3.9 – An elderly woman with aching shoulders and thighs, a painful temporal headache and a sudden onset of sight loss in her right eye.

A 73-year-old woman describes a 3-week history of stiffness in her proximal arms and thighs, which have become increasingly painful. The pain is especially bad at night and first thing in the morning. In the last 2 days she has noticed tenderness in the scalp when combing her hair and headache over the same site. Today she awoke to realize that she had no sight in her right eye.

▟▟ OSCE Counselling Case

OSCE COUNSELLING CASE 3.3 – 'Will having lupus give me problems should I want to become pregnant?'

Key concepts

In order to work through the core clinical cases in this chapter, you will need to understand the following key concepts.

The multi-system involvement of this group of conditions, although rare in routine practice, requires all clinicians to maintain awareness of them. Involvement of systems such as the kidneys and lungs can often be silent in the early stages, requiring active screening. Many of the differential diagnoses in this group will have similar investigation findings such as a high CRP and a positive antinuclear antibody (ANA), which can be found in infection and malignancy.

The connective tissue disorders are a group of conditions including rheumatoid arthritis, systemic lupus erythematosus (SLE), Sjögren's syndrome, myositis/dermatomyositis, scleroderma and undifferentiated connective tissue disease. Although recognizably different, they share many features and should be screened for as a group.

The vasculitides are a diverse group of conditions, which can be primary, or secondary in nature. The primary or systemic vasculitides are usually classified on the basis of the size of the arteries involved:

- Large vessel: temporal and Takayasu's vasculitis

- Medium sized: polyarteritis nodosa and Kawasaki's disease

- Small vessel: Wegener's granulomatosis, Churg–Strauss syndrome, microscopic polyarteritis, Henoch–Schönlein purpura, essential cryoglobulinaemic vasculitis and leukocytoclastic vasculitis.

Secondary causes include the connective tissue diseases, infection, malignancy and allergy, e.g. drug induced.

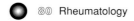

Answers

 CASE 3.7 – A young woman with joint pains and feeling unwell.

 Q1: What is the likely differential diagnosis?

A1

With a symmetrical small and large joint arthritis, a systemic illness including pleurisy and a facial rash, in a woman, SLE (lupus) is a possible diagnosis. Consider infection, sarcoid, vasculitis and malignancy.

 Q2: How would you investigate this case?

A2

A routine blood screen including FBC, ESR, U&Es and LFTs should be ordered, as well as ANA, double-stranded DNA (dsDNA) and antibodies to extractable nuclear antigen (ENA). Urinalysis looking for blood or protein should be checked. In view of the previous chest symptoms a chest radiograph should be ordered.

 Q3: How would you confirm the likely diagnosis?

A3

Finding a positive ANA rarely leads to a diagnosis of lupus. The diagnosis, like much of rheumatology, is clinical and a specialist opinion usually needs to be sought to confirm it. Often the American College of Rheumatology (ACR) revised diagnostic criteria are used as a basis to establish the diagnosis, which requires having 4 out of a list of 11 typical features of the condition. Lupus is also diagnosed by demonstrating typical histological features especially when patients do not fulfil the ACR.

 Q4: How would you initially manage the case?

A4

Once the diagnosis has been confirmed the management depends on the extent of systemic involvement, e.g. active lupus nephritis will require more aggressive management initially than someone who just has mild arthritis and a rash. Isolated rash and arthritis can be managed with NSAIDs, hydroxychloroquine and sun block. Systemically ill patients often require prednisolone, usually combined with immunosuppressive drugs to control their disease.

Q5: What are the principles of long-term management?

A5

The management of lupus requires a broad range of clinical skills and may require input from several disciplines. Complex cases are best managed by clinicians with experience of the condition. Lupus can affect any system in the body and any new symptoms should be investigated to check for possible lupus involvement. Renal, lung and cardiovascular involvement need to be regularly screened for. The use of toxic therapies can complicate matters with side effects. There is also an increased risk of infection as a result of the immunosuppressing nature of SLE and its treatments. In a young woman future pregnancies may well need careful planning because the disease and drugs may adversely affect fertility. Pregnancy can impose additional strains on already damaged organs such as the lungs or kidneys.

 Q6: What is the prognosis?

A6

Spontaneous remission or cure is unlikely. The prognosis of lupus depends on the severity of the condition and is particularly influenced by the presence of absence of renal disease with only 60 per cent of patients with renal disease being alive after 15 years.

 CASE 3.8 – 'You've seen me before with sinusitis. Now I feel terrible, my eye is sore and I think I coughed up blood today.'

 Q1: What is the likely differential diagnosis?

A1

With renal, upper and lower respiratory symptoms, eye inflammation, myalgia and arthralgia, and blood evidence of inflammation, systemic vasculitis is probable and in this case Wegener's granulomatosis is the most likely subtype. Alternative diagnoses such as malignancy need to be positively ruled out.

 Q2: How would you investigate this case?

A2

Tests should aim to assess the cause, extent and severity of the involvement. FBC, ESR, U&Es and LFTs may all demonstrate abnormal results. Sinus radiograph, chest radiograph, 24-hour urine protein loss and urine microscopy should also be performed. ANAs, complements C3, C4 and ANCA (anti-neutrophil cytoplasmic antigen) will help establish the diagnosis. Specialist ophthalmological and ear, nose and throat (ENT) assessment and treatment may be helpful.

 Q3: How would you confirm the likely diagnosis?

A3

Treatment of vasculitis is long term and typically requires long-term toxic therapy; therefore biopsy is regarded as the gold standard for diagnosis. The nasal mucosa, lung and kidney are possible sites for biopsy. A positive cANCA/PR3 result is highly specific and sensitive for Wegener's granulomatosis.

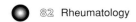

 Q4: How would you initially manage the case?

A4

Having assessed the extent of involvement, treatment typically involves an induction phase designed to arrest inflammation and a longer-term treatment phase aimed at maintaining disease suppression. Drugs commonly used are steroids, immunosuppressants and cytotoxics. Co-trimoxazole is prescribed for those patients with *Staphylococcus aureus* in their noses, because it is believed to reduce relapses of the condition when used in combination with other immunosuppressants.

 Q5: What are the principles of long-term management?

A5

In this patient with renal involvement, potential renal failure needs to be assessed. The lung involvement can progress to fibrosis. Involvement of the upper airways can produce aggressive local damage, even eroding through the floor of the anterior skull. Untreated eye involvement can lead to blindness. Secondary infection is a constant threat as a result of the condition and/or treatment. Flare-ups are not uncommon, often requiring temporary increases in treatment.

 Q6: What is the prognosis?

A6

A medical cure is not possible. Long-term follow-up with careful multi-system assessment is essential to maximize the success of treatment. The prognosis is adversely affected by renal involvement; overall the 10-year survival rate is about 80 per cent.

 CASE 3. 9 – An elderly woman with aching shoulders and thighs, a painful temporal headache and a sudden onset of sight loss in her right eye.

 Q1: What is the likely differential diagnosis?

A1

The history of polymyalgic symptoms, temporal headache and sudden onset of blindness strongly suggest a diagnosis of temporal arteritis.

 Q2: How would you investigate this case?

A2

This is a rare example of a rheumatological emergency. Consideration should be given to whether ordering tests will delay the introduction of prednisolone. After just 48 hours of prednisolone therapy the typical blood findings of a highly raised

ESR and the characteristic biopsy evidence will disappear. However, prompt initiation of steroids may promote return of vision in the affected eye and should preserve vision in the non-affected eye.

 Q3: How would you confirm the likely diagnosis?

A3

The definitive test is biopsy of an affected temporal artery. As a result of the irregular pattern of vessel involvement, single biopsy may be falsely negative in up to 30 per cent of cases.

 Q4: How would you initially manage the case?

A4

The initial management involves high-dose prednisolone, typically 40 mg/day or more. As treatment will last for more than 3 months, she should be commenced on bone protection therapy with a bisphosphonate and calcium and vitamin D_3.

 Q5: What are the principles of long-term management?

A5

The longer-term management involves reducing the steroids, balancing them against the recurrence of symptoms such as headache and proximal myalgia and a raised ESR. Most patients will eventually be able to come off steroids. If it is not possible to reduce the maintenance steroid dose, it may be necessary to commence steroid-sparing drugs such as azathioprine or methotrexate.

 Q6: What is the prognosis?

A6

Blindness occurs in up to 15 per cent of patients with this condition. The mortality is not raised compared with a matched population, even though aortic aneurysm, and cerebral and myocardial infarction are rare complications of this condition.

👥 OSCE Counselling Case – Answer

OSCE COUNSELLING CASE 3.3 – 'Will having lupus give me problems should I want to become pregnant?'

Having lupus can affect pregnancy in a number of ways. Overall lupus increases the risk of a conception not progressing to term from the normal 10 per cent to 25 per cent. Antiphospholipid antibody syndrome increases the risk of miscarriage. Those women who have Ro and La antibody-associated lupus have an approximately 5 per cent chance of transplacental spread of antibodies, producing neonatal lupus that can include neonatal heart block. Renal and pulmonary disease can be complicated by pregnancy. Finally many of the drugs used to treat lupus may adversely affect fertility.

BACK PAIN

? **Questions for each of the clinical case scenarios given**

Q1: What is the likely differential diagnosis?
Q2: How would you investigate this case?
Q3: How would you confirm the likely diagnosis?
Q4: How would you initially manage the case?
Q5: What are the principles of long-term management?
Q6: What is the prognosis?

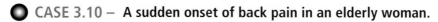

Clinical cases

● CASE 3.10 – A sudden onset of back pain in an elderly woman.

A 72-year-old woman describes an acute onset of mid-back pain. She has not had anything like this before and presents to the accident and emergency department (A&E). There was no obvious precipitant for her back problem. A radiograph reveals a wedge fracture of T8.

● CASE 3.11 – A stiff painful back and a red eye.

An ophthalmologist recommends a 26-year-old man to seek an opinion about his long history of back pain and stiffness after developing a red and painful left eye.

ŤŤ OSCE Counselling Case

OSCE COUNSELLING CASE 3.4 – 'What can I do to prevent osteoporotic fractures in the future?'

☞ Key concepts

In order to work through the core clinical cases in this chapter, you will need to understand the following key concepts.

Most adults will suffer back pain at some stage and for many this is a chronic problem. For this group reassurance, active support and advice to mobilize early and not expect a complete cure are important if disability is to be avoided. Patients under the age of 25 or over the age of 55 years who present with constant back pain of longer than 6 weeks' duration usually require radiological assessment. A history of malignancy, pain that wakes the patient, demonstrable motor weakness, bowel or bladder involvement and associated systemic involvement suggest significant pathology which may require more than just a simple radiograph.

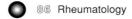

Answers

 CASE 3.10 – **A sudden onset of back pain in an elderly woman.**

 Q1: **What is the likely differential diagnosis?**

A1

A spontaneous osteoporotic fracture of the spine is the probable diagnosis. Other causes of a fracture include trauma, infection and malignancy. Women generally have a lower bone stock than men and with increasing age are prone to develop osteoporosis. The condition can be secondary to a number of medical conditions, including chronic obstructive pulmonary disease (COPD), malabsorption, inflammatory arthritis, steroid use, premature menopause, hyperparathyroidism, hyperthyroidism, chronic renal failure, immobility and autoimmune arthritis.

 Q2: **How would you investigate this case?**

A2

A history should be taken to look for the above risk factors, as well as for a past history of other low trauma fractures. Blood testing should be normal in primary osteoporosis but it is important to rule out secondary causes of osteoporosis and alternative diagnoses.

 Q3: **How would you confirm the likely diagnosis?**

A3

The gold standard for diagnosis is a dual energy X-ray absorptiometry (DEXA) scan of the lumbar spine and hip. Other techniques exist, including qualitative computed tomography (QCT), peripheral DEXA scan and ultrasonography of the heel. A DEXA scan of the spine and hip is best at predicting hip fracture and is sensitive and specific enough to allow monitoring of therapy. In this case provided that no alternative diagnoses are present, it is not necessary to scan this woman in order to justify starting medication.

Q4: **How would you initially manage the case?**

A4

Pain control is the first goal of management. Typically this will require opiate-based treatment and advice about rest. The pain normally settles progressively over a 12-week period. Calcitonin injections can be used in the first week after a fracture to augment pain control. The use of transcutaneous electronerve stimulation can augment pain control. Surgery, although still at an early stage of development, can be used to rebuild the vertebrae and reduce pain.

Q5: What are the principles of long-term management?

A5

The fracture, although painful, rarely produces neurological deficit. The principal risk is that having one osteoporotic fracture is a strong risk fracture for future fractures. Further vertebral fracture can produce a fixed kyphosis. Fracture of the hip is the most serious of the osteoporosis-associated fractures; up to one-third may die and only one-third will return to an independent existence after the fracture. Treatment involves bisphosphonates and usually calcium and vitamin D_3. Further fractures despite appropriate treatment with bisphosphonates may require treatment with teriparatide, a parathyroid hormone (PTH) analogue.

 Q6: What is the prognosis?

A6

Treatment of osteoporosis needs to be linked to a falls prevention strategy to maximize the longer-term outlook.

● CASE 3.11 − A stiff painful back and a red eye.

 Q1: What is the likely differential diagnosis?

A1

The connection to make is iritis and ankylosing spondylitis. It is possible that no connection exists, in which case in a young person the cause of the back pain could be mechanical, post-traumatic, associated with disc disease or developmental.

 Q2: How would you investigate this case?

A2

A blood screen may demonstrate raised inflammatory markers. A radiograph may demonstrate sclerosis and erosion of the sacro-iliac joint and squaring of the vertebrae with calcification of the intervertebral ligaments. Magnetic resonance imaging (MRI) can demonstrate changes not visible on a radiograph. An isotope bone scan can detect inflammation in the sacroiliac joint or lower back.

✓ Q3: How would you confirm the likely diagnosis?

A3

Demonstration of the typical radiological changes, although not present in every case, is diagnostic. The presence of the human leukocyte antigen HLA-B27 gene is not diagnostic because it is found in at least 7 per cent of the general population. Its absence, however, virtually rules out ankylosing spondylitis.

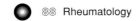

Q4: How would you initially manage the case?

A4

The principal mode of treatment of mild-to-moderate forms of the disease is physiotherapy. This can be augmented by NSAIDs; phenylbutazone, banned from general use, still has a place for pain relief in this condition. Methotrexate and sulphasalazine, although helpful for peripheral disease, do not influence axial disease significantly More aggressive ankylosing spondylitis not responding to the above measures can be treated with anti-TNF therapies.

Q5: What are the principles of long-term management?

A5

The more the spine is involved in ankylosis, the more complications can occur, including the mechanical effects of kyphosis or ankylosis of the ribs producing respiratory restriction, and a risk of fracture as a result of associated osteoporosis and the altered mechanics of the stiff spine. It is possible to develop an associated peripheral arthritis as well as psoriasis, iritis, colitis and inflammation of the genitourinary tract. Rarely, associated cardiac and pulmonary complications can occur.

Q6: What is the prognosis?

A6

Long-term surveillance aims to detect early the complications of this chronic illness. An essential part of follow-up also involves the monitoring of compliance with physiotherapy. The prognosis is adversely affected by age of onset below 16, early hip involvement, raised CRP and peripheral joint involvement.

♀♀ OSCE Counselling Case – Answer

OSCE COUNSELLING CASE 3.4 – 'What can I do to prevent osteoporotic fractures in the future?'

About 70 per cent of the risk of developing osteoporosis is genetic; however, a number of factors are important. Lifestyle measures such as refraining from smoking, keeping alcohol consumption within recommended limits and maintaining a healthy body mass index (BMI) will be beneficial. Calcium intake equivalent to 800 mg/day is important throughout adult life. The use of vitamin D_3 supplementation in frail elderly individuals is associated with a reduced incidence of hip fractures. Levels of exercise in childhood and adolescence are one of the determining factors of peak bone mass. In later life regular exercise will reduce bone loss and decrease the incidence of falls. In elderly, at-risk patients the use of hip protectors also reduces the incidence of hip fractures. Premature menopause is a risk factor for osteoporosis and the use of hormone replacement therapy (HRT) does delay the onset of menopausal bone loss until it is stopped. This translates into a lifetime fracture reduction risk of about 3 per cent. In those with risk factors, a DEXA scan can be used to assess bone density and appropriate therapy can reduce the risk of future fracture.

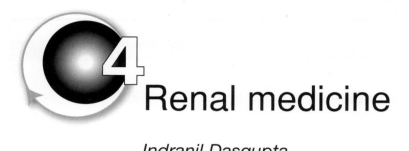

4 Renal medicine

Indranil Dasgupta

RENAL CASE STUDIES

? Questions for each of the clinical case scenarios given

Q1: What is the likely diagnosis?
Q2: How would you investigate this case?
Q3: How would you manage the case?
Q4: What is the prognosis?

Clinical cases

● CASE 4.1 – A 58-year-old man presenting with raised serum creatinine.

A 58-year-old South Asian man has recently been found to have a raised serum creatinine of 156 μmol/L (reference range: 60–120 μmol/L). He has been on antihypertensive treatment for 10 years and a smoker for 40 years. He is on nifedipine, atenolol and simvastatin. His serum creatinine was 121 μmol/L a year ago.

● CASE 4.2 – A 22-year-old woman presenting with progressive swelling of legs.

A 22-year-old white woman presented to her GP with progressive swelling of her legs of 2 weeks' duration. She was otherwise asymptomatic. On examination, she had oedema up to both knees and her blood pressure (BP) was 120/70 mmHg. Urinalysis revealed +++ proteins but no blood; serum creatinine was 92 μmol/L and serum albumin 1.8 g/dL.

● CASE 4.3 – A 34-year-old man presenting with microscopic haematuria.

A 34-year-old man was found to have microscopic haematuria on an insurance medical examination. He was asymptomatic. His BP was 124/80 mmHg and his serum creatinine 102 μmol/L.

● CASE 4.4 – A 62-year-old woman presenting with a raised serum creatinine, microscopic haematuria and proteinuria.

A 62-year-old woman presented to her GP with symptoms of tiredness, lethargy, aching joints, poor appetite and nausea of 4–6 weeks' duration. Physical examination was unremarkable except pallor and a BP of 160/100 mmHg. Routine blood tests revealed: haemoglobin (Hb) 10 g/dL, blood urea 26 mmol/L and serum creatinine 386 μmol/L (glomerular filtration rate or GFR 14 mL/min). The patient was referred to the local hospital. Further examination revealed purpuric spots in both legs and +++ blood and +++ protein on urinalysis.

● CASE 4.5 – A 76-year-old man presenting with dysuria and nocturia.

A 76-year-old man presented to his GP with a history of difficulty in passing urine in the form of hesitancy, poor stream and occasional pain while passing urine of 3 months' duration. He also suffered from nocturia. Physical examination was unremarkable. Urinalysis showed presence of + for each of blood and protein. Blood test showed a raised serum creatinine of 560 µmol/L (GFR 11 mL/min). The patient was urgently referred to the nearby district general hospital. Further examination in the hospital revealed a palpable bladder and a smoothly enlarged prostate on per rectal examination.

👥 OSCE Counselling Cases

OSCE COUNSELLING CASE 4.1 – **'I have recently been diagnosed as having chronic kidney disease. What problems can I expect to have?'**

OSCE COUNSELLING CASE 4.2 – **'As a patient with chronic kidney disease, do I have a higher risk of heart disease?'**

OSCE COUNSELLING CASE 4.3 – **'As a patient with chronic kidney disease, do I need to avoid any drugs?'**

OSCE COUNSELLING CASE 4.4 – **'As a patient with kidney failure, do I need to stick to a diet?'**

OSCE COUNSELLING CASE 4.5 – **'If I need to go on dialysis treatment what are the treatment options?'**

🔑 Key concepts

In order to work through the core clinical cases in this chapter, you will need to understand the following key concepts.

Common causes of end-stage renal failure

Diabetes is the most common cause of end-stage renal failure (ESRF) accounting for about 20 per cent of cases in England and Wales (nearly 50 per cent in the USA). The other main causes are glomerulonephritis (10 per cent), pyelonephritis (6.5 per cent), renovascular disease (7 per cent), hypertension (6 per cent) and adult polycystic kidney disease (PCK) (6 per cent) (Ansell D, Feest T, eds (2003) UK Renal Registry Report. Bristol: UK Renal Registry). In a good number of patients (nearly a quarter of patients in England and Wales), the aetiology is uncertain because these patients present late when it is difficult to establish a primary renal diagnosis.

Formulae for calculating creatinine clearance and GFR

Cockroft–Gault formula or creatinine clearance (mL/min):

Males: $= [1.23 \times (140 - \text{Age}) \times \text{Weight}]/[\text{Creatinine}]$.

Females: $[1.04 \times (140 - \text{Age}) \times \text{Weight}]/[\text{Creatinine}]$.

MDRD formula (abbreviated form: GFR in mL/min per 1.73 m²:

Males: GFR = 186 × ([Creatinine]/88.4)$^{-1.154}$ × Age$^{-0.203}$.

Females: GFR = 138 × ([Creatinine]/88.4)$^{-1.154}$ × Age$^{-0.203}$.

Multiply by 1.21 if the patient is African–Caribbean.

The MDRD formula is derived from Modification of Diet in Renal Disease study results.

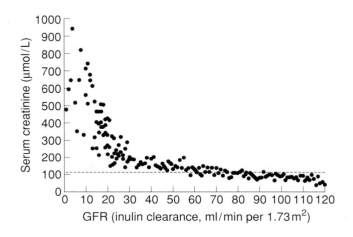

Figure 4.1 Relationship between serum creatinine and glomerular filtration rate (GFR). Serum creatinine remains normal until the GFR is around 60 mL/min.

Table 4.1 Stages of chronic kidney disease – NKF K/DOQI[a] classification

Stage	GFR (mL/min per 1.73 m²)	Description
1	≥ 90	Kidney damage with normal or high GFR
2	60–89	Mild
3	59–30	Moderate
4	29–15	Severe
5	< 15	End-stage kidney failure or on dialysis

[a]National Kidney Foundation, Kidney Disease Outcomes Quality Initiative.
GFR, glomerular filtration rate.

Reproduced with kind permission from the National Kidney Foundation (2002). K/DOQI Clinical Practice Guidelines for Chronic Kidney Disease: Evaluation, Classification and Stratification. *Ann J Kidney Dis* **39**: 19.

Answers

 CASE 4.1 – A 58-year-old man presenting with raised serum creatinine.

 Q1: What is the likely diagnosis?

A1

Chronic renal failure (CRF) – although this patient's serum creatinine was just outside the normal range a year ago, his calculated GFR using the MDRD formula was 57 mL/min and his current GFR is 40 mL/min. Serum creatinine is not a reliable test to assess renal function because it is influenced by a number of factors including age, muscle mass, renal tubular secretion and extrarenal loss of creatinine. A number of regression equations, which can predict GFR/creatinine clearance, are available and, of these, the Cockroft–Gault and MDRD are most commonly used.

The cause of CRF, in this case, is uncertain pending further investigations, although hypertensive nephrosclerosis is a possibility.

 Q2: How would you investigate this case?

A2

Urinalysis, full blood count (FBC), serum calcium and phosphate, immunology and renal ultrasonography would be the initial investigations. A low Hb, high serum phosphate and bilateral small kidneys on ultrasonography will support the diagnosis. Normal sized kidneys with significant microscopic haematuria and proteinuria, with or without a positive immunological test, will indicate the need for a renal biopsy to establish an underlying cause of the CRF.

 Q3: How would you manage the case?

A3

This patient suffers from moderate chronic kidney disease (CKD stage 3). Hypertension and proteinuria are the two most important progression promoters. Aggressive BP control is the most important measure to prevent/slow down progression of renal disease to ESRF. Target BP should be 130/80 mmHg. In patients with proteinuria > 1 g/ day, the target BP should be 125/75 mmHg. Angiotensin-converting enzyme (ACE) inhibitors and angiotensin receptor blockers reduce proteinuria, and have been shown to retard progression of renal disease. These patients are also at very high cardiovascular risk. They should be urged to stop smoking, lose weight if obese and be treated for hyperlipidaemia. Patient should also be advised to avoid non-steroidal anti-inflammatory and other nephrotoxic drugs.

 Q4: What is the prognosis?

A4

Chronic kidney disease in this patient is likely to progress to ESRF requiring dialysis or renal transplantation. Patients with CKD stage 3 have a significantly increased risk of cardiovascular morbidity and mortality.

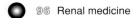 **CASE 4.2 – A 22-year-old woman presenting with progressive swelling of legs.**

 Q1: What is the likely diagnosis?

A1

Nephrotic syndrome – defined as the presence of oedema, heavy proteinuria (> 3 g/day) and hypoalbuminaemia with or without hypercholesterolaemia and hypertension.

The most common cause of nephrotic syndrome is minimal change nephropathy, especially in children. In adults, membranous nephropathy and focal segmental glomerulosclerosis (FSGS) are also common causes of nephrotic syndrome. In as many as 30 per cent of cases nephrotic syndrome is the result of a systemic disease such as diabetes mellitus, systemic lupus erythematosus (SLE), amyloidosis, multiple myeloma.

 Q2: How would you investigate this case?

A2

Refer to a nephrologist for a renal biopsy. Blood sugar and lipids should be checked. Blood should be sent off for immunological tests such as antinuclear antibodies, complements, serum immunoglobulins and cryoglobulins.

 Q3: How would you manage the case?

A3

Management depends on renal biopsy finding. Minimal change disease is treated with high-dose prednisolone (1 mg/kg, maximum 80 mg/day). This is continued until 1 week after remission (may take up to 16 weeks). The dose is then reduced gradually with a view to stop between 8 and 12 weeks. FSGS sometimes responds to a prolonged course of corticosteroids. Oedema is treated with salt restriction and loop diuretics. Severely nephrotic patients are treated with heparin while they are admitted to hospital to prevent venous thromboembolism. ACE inhibitors are often used to treat hypertension and reduce proteinuria. Hypercholesterolaemia should be treated with a statin.

Q4: What is the prognosis?

A4

Minimal change nephrotic syndrome in children responds promptly to high-dose corticosteroid therapy. In adults, it does not always respond to corticosteroids as quickly and often relapses. Membranous nephropathy spontaneously remits in up to 25 per cent of patients and progresses to ESRF in about 40 per cent of patients at 15 years. FSGS leads to ESRF in about 50 per cent of cases and often recurs after transplantation.

CASE 4.3 – A 34-year-old man presenting with microscopic haematuria.

 Q1: What is the likely diagnosis?

A1

Isolated microscopic haematuria – the most common causes of this in young people are IgA nephropathy and thin basement membrane disease. IgA nephropathy is the most common form of glomerulonephritis characterized by deposition of IgA in the mesangium. Thin basement membrane disease is a familial condition, which is characterized by uniform thinning of the glomerular basement membrane. The other causes of microscopic haematuria are stones, cystic diseases of kidney, tumour and inflammatory diseases of the urinary tract. Urological causes predominate in older patients.

 Q2: How would you investigate this case?

A2

Urinalysis needs to be repeated, because transient microscopic haematuria may not be significant. Moreover, presence of significant proteinuria (++ or more) may signify a more aggressive form of glomerulonephritis. Ideally, urine should be sent for microscopy to ensure there are two or more red blood cells (RBCs) per high power field. Dipsticks are very sensitive and often detect less significant haematuria, Hb and myoglobin. Ultrasonography of the kidneys and urinary tracts should be done to exclude a macroscopic pathology. Serum immunoglobulins, complements, autoantibodies and ANCA (anti-neutrophil cytoplasmic antigen) should be checked. A raised serum IgA level will support a diagnosis of IgA nephropathy. Normal autoantibody, complement and ANCA tests will make an underlying autoimmune disease or vasculitis unlikely. If there is significant proteinuria (> 1 g/day) a renal biopsy will be indicated to exclude acute glomerulonephritis.

 Q3: How would you manage the case?

A3

No specific treatment is indicated. The patient should be followed on a regular basis – perhaps annually – for measurement of BP, urinalysis and serum creatinine. Should the patient develop significant proteinuria or there is a rise in serum creatinine, renal biopsy should be considered. If the patient develops hypertension, it should be treated, preferably with an ACE inhibitor.

 Q4: What is the prognosis?

A4

Prognosis is good. IgA nephropathy rarely progresses to advanced renal failure in the absence of significant proteinuria, hypertension and/ or raised serum creatinine at presentation. Thin basement membrane disease rarely causes proteinuria, renal impairment or hypertension.

CASE 4.4 – A 62-year-old woman presenting with a raised serum creatinine, microscopic haematuria and proteinuria.

 Q1: What is the likely diagnosis?

A1

Acute glomerulonephritis, possibly associated with systemic vasculitis.

 Q2: How would you investigate this case?

A2

Urine microscopy – presence of RBC casts – will support the diagnosis of acute glomerulonephritis. Send off blood for immunological tests such as ANCA, anti-GBM (glomerular basement membrane) antibodies, antinuclear antibodies (ANAs), immunoglobulins and complements. A positive ANCA test will support a diagnosis of systemic vasculitis (cytoplasmic or cANCA is associated with Wegener's granulomatosis and perinuclear or pANCA with microscopic polyangiitis). A positive ANA (especially anti-double-stranded [anti-dsDNA]) with low complements will support a diagnosis of lupus nephritis. Raised anti-GBM antibody titre will raise the suspicion of Goodpasture's disease. Chest radiograph should be performed to look for consolidation, cavitation or pulmonary haemorrhage, which supports a diagnosis of either systemic vasculitis or anti-GBM disease. Ultrasonography of kidneys. Renal biopsy will confirm the diagnosis of acute glomerulonephritis.

 Q3: How would you manage the case?

A3

Immunosuppressive treatment is initiated after confirmation of diagnosis by a renal biopsy. However, if the patient is too ill to biopsy, a presumptive diagnosis is made based on clinical features and positive ANCA test. The standard immunosuppressive regimen consists of oral prednisolone (1 mg/kg per day, maximum 80 mg/day) and cyclophosphamide (2 mg/kg per day). Intravenous pulsed methylprednisolone and/or plasma exchange is used for induction of remission in patients with aggressive (life- or organ-threatening) disease. After 2 weeks, the dose of prednisolone is reduced gradually to 15 mg at 3 months and 10 mg at 6 months. To minimize side effects with prolonged use, cyclophosphamide is changed after 3 months to azathioprine for maintenance treatment. In view of the risk of relapse (30–50 per cent at 3–5 years), maintenance treatment using small doses of prednisolone and azathioprine is often continued long term.

 Q4: What is the prognosis?

A4

Untreated systemic vasculitis is associated with high mortality rate (90 per cent at 2 years). Immunosuppressive treatment, as described above, leads to control of disease in 80–90 per cent of patients. Pulmonary haemorrhage and dialysis dependence at presentation are poor prognostic features. As a rule, patients who require dialysis treatment at presentation are less likely to have significant improvement in their kidney function.

CASE 4.5 – A 76-year-old man presenting with dysuria and nocturia.

 Q1: What is the likely diagnosis?

A1

Acute or acute-on-chronic renal impairment resulting from bladder neck obstruction by an enlarged prostate.

 Q2: How would you investigate this case?

A2

- Urinary catheterization: a large residual volume of urine would confirm the diagnosis of urinary retention caused by bladder neck obstruction. Ultrasonography of the abdomen and pelvis would reveal bilateral hydronephrosis, hydroureter and an enlarged prostate. Bilateral small kidneys or cortical thinning would suggest that the obstruction (chronic retention) is long standing.

- Serum prostate-specific antigen (PSA) assay: a high serum concentration would suggest possible prostatic malignancy (caution: sample taken after per rectal examination/catheterization may show a spuriously high level).

 Q3: How would you manage the case?

A3

Immediate bladder catheterization should be done to relieve obstruction. If catheterization is difficult, the urology team should be informed, because suprapubic catheterization may be required. Fluid balance (intake and output) should be monitored, because the patient is likely to have a large diuresis. Urea and electrolytes should also be monitored daily. If the patient is unable to drink a large amount of fluid to keep up with the urine output, intravenous fluid – 0.9 per cent saline with or without potassium chloride depending on serum potassium level – should be infused. When the renal function stabilizes, the urology team should be involved for long-term management of prostatic enlargement. Occasionally, bilateral nephrostomy drainage is required if there is no significant diuresis after bladder catheterization and/or no significant improvement in hydronephrosis on repeat ultrasonography.

 Q4: What is the prognosis?

A4

This depends on the chronicity of urinary obstruction. In most cases, renal function improves significantly and remains stable for many years. In patients who have long-standing chronic obstruction, especially those who have very thin renal cortex on ultrasonography, renal function may not improve at all. These patients go on to need dialysis treatment.

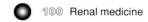

᚛ᚂᚃ OSCE Counselling Cases – Answers

OSCE COUNSELLING CASE 4.1 – 'I have recently been diagnosed as having chronic kidney disease. What problems can I expect to have?'

Mild or moderate CKD (GFR > 30 mL/min) does not generally cause any symptoms. In severe CKD (GFR < 30 mL/min), common symptoms are tiredness and generalized itching. As dialysis approaches, patients develop anorexia, nausea and vomiting. These 'uraemic symptoms' are the result of progressive accumulation of waste products (uraemic toxins) and anaemia.

The following are the common complications of CKD.

ANAEMIA

It results mainly from a low concentration erythropoietin. The other factors that contribute to anaemia in CKD are functional iron deficiency, anaemia of chronic disease, upper gastrointestinal (GI) blood loss and direct suppression of bone marrow by the waste products. The patient is treated with erythropoietin injection when Hb drops below 11 g/dL provided there is no iron deficiency.

SALT AND FLUID RETENTION

This leads to oedema, hypertension and, in severe cases, pulmonary oedema. The patients are advised to restrict salt and fluid intake, and treated with loop diuretics.

HYPERTENSION

This is common and strict BP control is needed to slow down or prevent deterioration of kidney function. The target BP is 130/80 mmHg. The ACE inhibitors and angiotensin receptor blockers are particularly beneficial in terms of protection of renal function.

RENAL BONE DISEASE OR OSTEODYSTROPHY

This is not a single entity. It comprises secondary hyperparathyroidism, adynamic bone disease (resulting from low bone turnover), osteomalacia or a combination of these. Phosphate retention and diminished production of active vitamin D (caused by impaired 1α-hydroxylation) are the initiating events. The patients are advised to follow a low-phosphate diet from an early stage and put on phosphate binders such as calcium carbonate and acetate. They are also treated with α-hydroxylated vitamin D (such as alfacalcidol) if their serum parathyroid hormone (PTH) concentration is high.

CARDIOVASCULAR DISEASE

Patients with CKD have a very high risk of heart disease and strokes. This is discussed in detail on page 101.

MALNUTRITION

This occurs as a result of a combination of anorexia with nausea/vomiting in the later stages of CKD and dietary restrictions imposed to tackle high serum phosphate and potassium. Most renal units employ dietitians who advise these patients regularly.

INFECTIONS

These are common because of reduced immunity as a result of a combination of impaired T-cell and neutrophil functions. The patients are immunized with hepatitis B vaccine at an early stage. It is also recommended that they have influenza immunization annually and pneumococcal vaccination 5-yearly.

OSCE COUNSELLING CASE 4.2 – 'As a patient with chronic kidney disease, do I have a higher risk of heart disease?'

Chronic kidney disease is associated with high cardiovascular risk. Patients with CKD have up to three fold risk of suffering cardiovascular events and death. Patients with ESRF who are on dialysis have even higher cardiovascular risk. Death as a result of cardiovascular disease is 10–20 times higher in dialysis patients compared with the general population.

Apart from the classic risk factors such as hypertension, hyperlipidaemia and smoking, these patients also have left ventricular hypertrophy, chronic anaemia, abnormal apolipoproteins, raised serum phosphate (with or without high calcium phosphate product), arterial calcification, elevated plasma homocysteine level, enhanced coagulability and abnormal endothelial function. All of these probably contribute towards their extremely high cardiovascular morbidity and mortality. It is, therefore, important to treat their blood pressure aggressively, urge them to stop smoking, and put them on aspirin and statin. The serum phosphate level is generally controlled with dietary restriction and the use of phosphate binders. Anaemia should be treated early and effectively with erythropoietin.

OSCE COUNSELLING CASE 4.3 – 'As a patient with chronic kidney disease, do I need to avoid any drugs?'

A variety of insults, which would have little impact on healthy kidneys, may cause significant loss of renal function in patients with pre-existing kidney damage. When more than one nephrotoxic factor is present, the risk of worsening renal function is much increased. Apart from renal disease itself, important predisposing factors include:

- Old age: GFR falls by 50 per cent by 80 years of age as a result of normal ageing processes
- Diabetes
- Atherosclerosis: peripheral vascular disease often involves the renal arteries too
- Cardiac failure: low cardiac output leads to 'pre-renal' uraemia
- Hypovolaemia
- Hepatic failure: associated with renal vasoconstriction and 'pre-renal' uraemia
- Myeloma: with or without hypercalcaemia or hyperuricaemia
- Transplant kidney: vulnerable even with a normal creatinine.

COMMON NEPHROTOXIC AGENTS

- ACE inhibitors and angiotensin receptor blockers: reduce GFR in renal arterial stenosis (RAS) and sometimes in chronic renal failure. Do not use if RAS is likely. Captopril is shorter acting and so more quickly reversible. Beware a major drop in BP in volume-depleted patients. Check creatinine before and 3–7 days after starting treatment. Watch K^+ also.
- Non-steroidal anti-inflammatory drugs (NSAIDs): reduce the vasodilatory effect of prostaglandins and lead to unopposed vasoconstriction.

- Aminoglycosides: trough and peak levels should be measured. The nephrotoxic effect may also be related to the total cumulative dose received.

- Ciclosporin: a dose-related NSAID-like effect.

- Radiological contrast: protection of GFR with adequate hydration pre-study is essential.

- Tetracyclines: doxycycline is metabolized in the liver and is the only safe one.

OSCE COUNSELLING CASE 4.4 – 'As a patient with kidney failure, do I need to stick to a diet?'

Most renal units have specialist renal dietitians attached to the unit. They advise patients regularly about their dietary and fluid restrictions. Patients with CRF need to restrict their phosphate intake at an early stage; recent guidelines suggest phosphate restriction when GFR drops to < 60 mL/min. Phosphate is found in almost all foods, but is especially high in milk and milk products, liver, dried beans and nuts. Dialysis does not clear phosphate very effectively and, therefore, the patient needs to continue on a low-phosphate diet even when on dialysis. Patients are also asked to restrict their potassium intake. Major sources of potassium are fruits (especially citrus fruits and bananas), vegetables, chocolate, coffee and salt substitutes. Salt restriction is recommended to help BP control and fluid retention even when the patient is on dialysis. Patients are advised to restrict their total fluid intake to about a litre a day unless they have a significant urine output.

OSCE COUNSELLING CASE 4.5 – 'If I need to go on dialysis treatment what are the treatment options?'

Renal replacement therapy (RRT) is generally required when the GFR is around 10 mL/min (ESRF). Most patients with CRF are symptomatic (with anorexia, nausea and vomiting) at this stage. Some advocate earlier start but, as yet, there is no convincing evidence to suggest a survival benefit of early commencement of dialysis. Patients with diabetes often become symptomatic at an earlier stage and start dialysis with a higher GFR compared with patients who do not have diabetes. Some CRF patients start dialysis as an emergency because of either intractable hyperkalaemia or severe pulmonary oedema.

There are three modalities of RRT:

1. Haemodialysis

2. Peritoneal dialysis – either continuous ambulatory (CAPD) or automated (APD)

3. Renal transplantation.

The optimal choice of modality of RRT depends on the patient's age, functional capacity, co-morbidities, family support and, above all, patient's choice. Some patients receive all three at various stages of their illness. Some patients, who have chosen not to have dialysis treatment or are deemed unlikely to benefit from it, are treated conservatively with full supportive treatment including erythropoietin therapy.

The annual acceptance rate and prevalence of RRT in the UK are 101 and 626 per million population respectively. Forty-six per cent of prevalent patients have a functioning transplant and 73 per cent of the dialysis patients are on haemodialysis (Ansell D, Feest T, eds (2003) UK Renal Registry Report. Bristol: UK Renal Registry).

RENAL EMERGENCIES

? Questions for each of the clinical case scenarios given

Q1: What is the likely diagnosis?
Q2: How would you investigate this case?
Q3: What would be the initial management?
Q4: What would be the long-term management?

Clinical cases

● CASE 4.6 – A 60-year-old man presented with diarrhoea, vomiting and renal impairment.

A 60-year-old man, previously fit and well, presented to the accident and emergency department (A&E) with a 1-week history of diarrhoea and vomiting. He was unwell and clammy, his skin turgor was poor, and his pulse and BP were 120/min and 80/60 mmHg, respectively. Initial investigations showed serum Na^+ 126 mmol/L, K^+ 3.0 mmol/L, urea 28 mmol/L and creatinine 306 μmol/L (calculated GFR 22.5 mL/min).

● CASE 4.7 – A 72-year-old man presenting with hyperkalaemia.

A 72-year-old man has been referred by the GP to A&E with a history of being non-specifically unwell for 2 days. He has a past history of ischaemic heart disease, atrial fibrillation, congestive cardiac failure and stable CRF. His regular medications include isosorbide mononitrate, digoxin, furosemide, spironolactone and an ACE inhibitor. On examination the patient is mildly confused, dehydrated, peripherally cold, bradycardic and hypotensive (BP 96/60 mmHg). His initial blood tests show Na^+ 130 mmol/L, K^+ 7.2 mmol/L, urea 42 mmol/L and creatinine of 412 μmol/L (GFR 14 mL/min).

● CASE 4.8 – A 68-year-old woman with CRF presenting with shortness of breath.

A 68-year-old woman, a known CRF patient, has presented to A&E with acute shortness of breath. Computer records suggest that her most recent serum creatinine from about a month earlier was 256 μmol/L (GFR 21 mL/min) and her regular medication includes furosemide 80 mg daily. She has recently been commenced on an NSAID for arthritis. On examination, she has oedema up to her mid-thighs, her jugular venous pressure (JVP) is raised at 6 cm, and there are crackles in both lung bases up to the midzones. Her admission ECG does not show any ischaemic changes, and her urea and electrolytes (U&Es) show: Na^+ 138 mmol/L, K^+ 5.6 mmol/L, urea 38 mmol/L, creatinine 446 μmol/L (GFR 12 mL/min).

● CASE 4.9 – A 34-year-old man presenting with severe hypertension and renal impairment.

A 34-year-old man of African–Caribbean origin has been referred by his GP for severe hypertension. On examination, his BP is 240/140 mmHg, he is slightly confused, there is mild pedal oedema, there are a few basal crackles and neurological examination is normal except for bilateral papilloedema. Urine analysis shows blood ++, protein ++. His Hb is 10.2 g/dL and U&Es show Na^+ 136 mmol/L, K^+ 3.0 mmol/L, urea 14 mmol/L and creatinine 206 μmol/L (GFR 54 mL/min).

🔑 Key concepts

In order to work through the core clinical cases in this chapter, you will need to understand the following key concepts.

Common causes of acute renal failure (ARF)

Pre-renal

As a result of ineffective perfusion of kidneys that are structurally normal

- Hypovolaemia: blood loss, GI loss, burns
- Low cardiac output states
- Shock
- Certain drugs: NSAIDs, ACE inhibitors

Renal

Structural damage to glomeruli and tubules

- Acute tubular necrosis (ATN): most common cause (45 per cent), results from prolonged hypoperfusion due to hypovolaemia (as above)
- Acute glomerulonephritis and vasculitis
- Acute interstitial nephritis: idiopathic, drugs, infection
- Vascular disease

Post-renal

As a result of urinary tract obstruction

- Prostatic hypertrophy
- Bladder tumour
- Gynaecological malignancy
- Neuropathic bladder.

Investigations to organize in ARF

Urine

Dipstick (blood and protein suggest acute glomerulonephritis), microscopy (RBC casts diagnostic of acute glomerulonephritis), urine electrolytes (to distinguish pre-renal from ATN)

Blood

- FBC, clotting: for disseminated intravascular coagulation (DIC), rarely haemolytic uraemic syndrome/TTP (thrombotic thrombocytopenic purpura)
- U&Es, Ca^{2+} and phosphate, glucose, creatine kinase (for rhabdomyolysis), CRP (for vascultis, sepsis)

- Immunology: autoantibodies (for SLE), ANCA (for vascultis), anti-GBM antibodies (for Goodpasture's syndrome), complements (low in SLE, infective endocarditis), immunoglobulins (for IgA nephropathy, myeloma)

- Blood cultures (sepsis, infective endocarditis), hepatitis B and C (in preparation for dialysis)

- ECG: for hyperkalaemic changes

- Chest radiograph: for pulmonary oedema, pneumonia

- Ultrasonography: to exclude obstruction.

Indications for urgent dialysis in ARF

- Severe hyperkalaemia (> 6.5 mmol/L or less with ECG changes, despite medical treatment)

- Pulmonary oedema

- Severe acidosis (pH < 7.1)

- Severe uraemia (vomiting, encephalopathy)

- Uraemic pericarditis

Overall mortality rate in ARF is about 50 per cent (up to 80 per cent in patients who require dialysis).

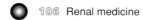

Answers

 CASE 4.6 – A 60-year-old man presented with diarrhoea, vomiting and renal impairment.

Q1: What is the likely diagnosis?

A1

Pre-renal failure or ATN resulting from reduced circulatory blood volume secondary to diarrhoea and vomiting. Loss of circulatory volume, caused by either salt and water depletion or haemorrhage, leads to reduced renal blood supply. This results in selective cortical vasoconstriction and oliguria (urine output < 400 mL/day). Initially this is reversible but when prolonged leads to ATN (ischaemic injury to the proximal tubular epithelial cells) and rarely to acute cortical necrosis

 Q2: How would you investigate this case?

A2

Urinalysis (dipstick test for blood and protein), urine microscopy, U&Es, FBC, serum bicarbonate, calcium and phosphate. Presence of significant amount of blood and protein (++ or more) in urine would raise a suspicion of acute glomerulonephritis. Urine Na^+ concentration of < 20 mmol/L would suggest reversible pre-renal failure, whereas > 40 mmol/L would suggest that ATN has set in. Low Hb and/ or a raised serum phosphate may indicate the presence of pre-existing chronic renal impairment.

 Q3: What would be the initial management?

A3

Intravenous access and intravenous infusion should be set up immediately. The ideal fluid replacement in this setting would be 0.9 per cent saline with potassium supplementation. In the presence of severe metabolic acidosis, sodium bicarbonate (1.26 per cent) infusion should be considered. It is preferable to remove the patient to a high dependency unit with a view to establishing central venous access to monitor central venous pressure (CVP). Pulse, BP and urine output should be monitored hourly. In the absence of CVP monitoring, lung bases should be auscultated frequently to prevent over-hydration leading to pulmonary oedema. Urea and electrolytes should be repeated in 4–6 hours to review progress.

 Q4: What would be the long-term management?

A4

Pre-renal failure is a rapidly reversible condition. In established ARF caused by ATN, it may take as long as 6 weeks for renal function to return to normal and the patient will require dialysis treatment for this period (1 per cent require long-term dialysis). If the patient is haemodynamically compromised, an initial period of continuous veno-venous haemofiltration (CVVH) may be necessary (generally in the intensive care unit [ICU]). If renal function does not improve within 24 hours, ultrasonography should be requested to exclude urinary tract obstruction. Small shrunken kidneys on ultrasonography would suggest that the patient has CRF.

 ## CASE 4.7 – A 72-year-old man presenting with hyperkalaemia.

 Q1: What is the likely diagnosis?

A1

Severe hyperkalaemia as a result of a combination of a potassium-sparing diuretic and an ACE inhibitor in the setting of chronic renal impairment. There is also a possible acute-on-chronic renal impairment caused by over-diuresis, as evidenced by a disproportionately high blood urea level and low Na^+.

 Q2: How would you investigate this case?

A2

A 12-lead ECG to see if there are any changes of hyperkalaemia – tall, peaked T waves, widening of QRS, reduction in height of P (may disappear) and R waves, sine wave pattern (pre-cardiac arrest).

 Q3: What would be the initial management?

A3

Severe hyperkalaemia (> 6.5 mmol/L) and the presence of ECG changes in this scenario warrant urgent treatment of hyperkalaemia as follows:

- Calcium gluconate: 10 mL 10 per cent i.v. over 5 min to counteract the adverse effect of hyperkalaemia on the cardiac conduction system (through a central line or a large cannula in a big vein to avoid delay).
- Infusion of 10 U insulin in 50 mL 50 per cent glucose i.v. through a pump over 30 min to drive K^+ into intracellular space.
- Nebulized salbutamol: 5 mg to help K^+ enter intracellular space.
- Sodium bicarbonate: 8.4 per cent 50 mL i.v. over 30 min – should be considered especially if acidotic (caution: may precipitate tetany if the serum Ca^{2+} is low).
- Calcium resonium 30 g rectally or 15 g orally to help exchange K^+ for Ca^{2+} in the gut.
- To check U&Es in 2 h and repeat glucose and insulin infusion and nebulized salbutamol if serum K^+ remains dangerously high (> 6.5 mmol/L) or ECG changes persist.
- If serum K^+ continues to remain > 6.5 mmol/mL or ECG changes persist despite treatment, haemodialysis may be required.

Intravenous infusion of 0.9 per cent saline to correct dehydration.

Q4: What would be the long-term management?

A4

The ACE inhibitor and spironolactone must be stopped. Refer the patient to the nephrologist for long-term management. If renal function returns to near the baseline, the ACE inhibitor may be restarted cautiously in the future if clinically indicated, i.e. poor left ventricular function on echocardiography. The patient should be followed up closely, preferably in the renal clinic.

● CASE 4.8 – A 68-year-old woman with CRF presenting with shortness of breath.

 Q1: What is the likely diagnosis?

A1

This patient's severe shortness of breath is likely to be caused by pulmonary oedema secondary to severe fluid retention. Acute deterioration in renal function has probably been precipitated by the recent introduction of an NSAID. NSAIDs reduce renal blood flow in patients with pre-existing renal disease and, thereby, cause deterioration of renal function. They can also cause acute interstitial nephritis leading to acute renal impairment.

 Q2: How would you investigate this case?

A2

Chest radiograph to confirm the diagnosis of pulmonary oedema (Figure 4.2). Arterial blood gas (ABG) analysis should be done to assess the degree of hypoxia, to ascertain whether there is any evidence of CO_2 retention and assess the degree of metabolic acidosis associated with renal failure.

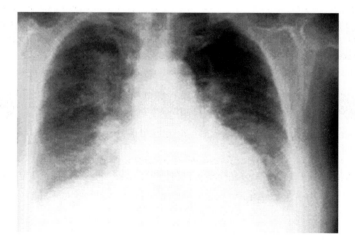

Figure 4.2 Chest radiograph for Case 4.8.

(This 'real' patient had a positive cANCA test and the renal biopsy showed the presence of acute necrotizing crescentic glomerulonephritis.)

Q3: What would be the initial management?

A3

Furosemide 80 mg i.v. If there is no significant diuresis, furosemide should be repeated using a higher dose (up to 250 mg i.v.). High-concentration oxygen should be given with a facemask. It may be necessary to use CPAP (continuous positive airway pressure) or even to ventilate the patient in the ITU if the patient is severely hypoxic. If the patient remains severely short of breath and oligo-anuric despite high-dose intravenous furosemide, the patient will need to be referred for urgent haemodialysis or haemofiltration.

 Q4: What would be the long-term management?

A4

Long-term management will depend on whether her renal function returns to baseline/near baseline after stopping the NSAID. If renal function improves, long-term management will consist of salt and fluid restriction, high-dose oral diuretic therapy and avoidance of nephrotoxic agents. The patient will need to be prepared for dialysis treatment. On the other hand, if her renal function fails to improve, she will require acute dialysis leading to long-term dialysis treatment.

 CASE 4.9 – A 34-year-old man presenting with severe hypertension and renal impairment.

 Q1: What is the likely diagnosis?

A1

Malignant hypertension, which is defined as severe hypertension, often > 200/140 mmHg; this is associated with papilloedema, usually accompanied by retinal haemorrhage and exudates, with or without renal impairment or neurological symptoms. It most commonly occurs in patients with long-standing uncontrolled hypertension. Differential diagnosis of this case scenario would be acute glomerulonephritis with severe hypertension.

 Q2: How would you investigate this case?

A2

A chest radiograph must be done to confirm or exclude pulmonary oedema. If confusion persists/deteriorates (deteriorating Glasgow Coma Score [GCS]), urgent computed tomography (CT) of the brain should be organized to exclude infarction or haemorrhage.

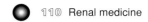
 Q3: What would be the initial management?

A3

Controlled lowering of blood pressure should be attempted with intravenous infusion of labetalol (a combined α- and β-adrenergic blocker) or sodium nitroprusside (a combined arteriolar and venodilator). The goal is to lower diastolic BP to between 100 and 105 mmHg, with systolic pressure around 160 mmHg, over 2–6 hours. Rapid lowering of BP may lead to cerebral vasospasm, resulting in cerebral infarction. The patient should ideally be treated in a high-dependency unit. If parenteral antihypertensive agents are not available, oral agents may be used but their use (especially sublingual nifedipine) is associated with the risk of causing excessive lowering of BP, leading to stroke or myocardial infarction.

 Q4: What would be the long-term management?

A4

Once the BP is controlled, the patient should be switched to oral antihypertensive therapy with gradual reduction of diastolic BP to 85–90 mmHg over 2–3 months. The patient should be investigated for a secondary cause of hypertension. Renal biopsy is indicated if renal function fails to stabilize with BP control. Long-term follow-up is needed for careful monitoring of renal function and strict control of BP because renal function may deteriorate progressively to ESRF.

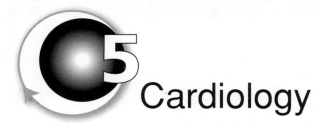

5 Cardiology

Nevianna Tomson and Neeraj Prasad

? **Questions for each of the clinical case scenarios given**

Q1: What specific questions would you ask the patient?
Q2: What is the most likely diagnosis?
Q3: What examination would you perform?
Q4: What would be the initial management?
Q5: What investigations would you request to confirm a diagnosis?
Q6: What other issues should be addressed?

Clinical cases

● CASE 5.1 – A 34-year-woman with palpitations.

A 34-year-old woman presented with a 3-hour history of palpitations. She is mildly dyspnoeic and has some chest pain. She has been feeling anxious and suffering from insomnia for the last few weeks. On direct questioning she admits to a 10-day history of diarrhoea. On examination she has a tachycardia and her pulse is irregular.

● CASE 5.2 – A 53-year-old man with sudden onset of chest pain.

A 53-year-old man is brought into the accident and emergency department (A&E) by ambulance complaining of sudden onset of severe central chest pain. He is cold and clammy, and appears breathless.

● CASE 5.3 – An 80-year-old patient collapses, requiring cardiopulmonary resuscitation (CPR).

A 80-year-old woman collapsed at home and has been brought into A&E unconscious. She was given basic life support at home by her daughter who happens to work as a ward sister on coronary care. The paramedics are performing CPR as the patient is wheeled into A&E accompanied by her tearful daughter.

● CASE 5.4 – A 65-year-old man with tearing chest pain.

A 65-year-old man was brought into A&E complaining of severe tearing pain between the shoulder blades. Initially the pain was extremely severe but has now mildly subsided to a dull ache in the chest. He is normally fit and well apart from hypertension, for which he has been seeing the GP.

● CASE 5.5 – A 25-year-old man with a heart murmur.

A 25-year-old man recently attended a medical in the process of getting into the police force. He has been told that he has a heart murmur.

♔♔ OSCE Counselling Cases

OSCE COUNSELLING CASE 5.1 – 'Can I stop my warfarin (anticoagulation in a patient with prosthetic heart valve)?'

A 24-year-old woman had a metal prosthetic heart valve inserted 4 years ago after a severe episode of bacterial endocarditis that degenerated her mitral valve. She has done very well since the surgery and has been on warfarin, regularly attending an anticoagulation clinic. She has come to see you today because she wants to have a family but has read on the internet that warfarin can damage the baby. Can she stop her warfarin?

OSCE COUNSELLING CASE 5.2 – The use of anti-anginal medication.

This 73-year-old man has recently been diagnosed with angina. He is able to walk 300 metres before experiencing chest tightness, but considerably less when there is an incline. His recent exercise stress test has indicated ischaemic heart disease (IHD) and he has been prescribed sublingual GTN (glyceryl trinitrate) tablets and a β-adrenoreceptor blocker. Please advise him on how to use the medication and explain any side effects of which he should be aware.

OSCE COUNSELLING CASE 5.3 – 'I have heart failure. Do I need to take my medications for life?'

A 65-year-old man with known IHD, hypertension and diabetes mellitus has recently been complaining of shortness of breath. An echocardiogram has confirmed left ventricular (LV) systolic dysfunction, which is moderately severe, and he has been started on ramipril 10 mg once daily, bisoprolol 2.5 mg once daily and spironolactone 25 mg once daily. He is very concerned about the number of medications that he is now on because these are additional to his other therapies. Explain the importance of his diagnosis and treatments to him.

☛ Key concepts

In order to work through the core clinical cases in this chapter, you will need to understand the following key concepts.

Benefits of drug management in chronic heart failure

- Diuretics: loop diuretics and thiazide diuretics improve symptoms of congestion.

- Spironolactone 25–50 mg once daily improves survival in severe (New York Heart Association [NYHA] stage III/IV) heart failure

- Angiotensin-converting enzyme (ACE) inhibitors: improved symptoms, exercise capacity and survival in patients with asymptomatic and symptomatic systolic dysfunction.

  – lisinopril 2.5 mg initial dose, 20 mg once daily target dose, sometimes up to 30 mg once daily

  – ramipril 1.25–2.5 mg initial dose, 10 mg once daily target dose

  – captopril* 6.25 mg initial dose, 50 mg three times daily target dose.

- Angiotensin II antagonists: treatment of symptomatic heart failure in patients intolerant to ACE inhibitors:*

    – losartan and valsartan

- β Blockers: improved symptoms and survival in stable patients who are already receiving ACE inhibitor with LV systolic dysfunction

    – Bisoprolol (Cardicor) 1.25 mg once daily titrated with close monitoring to 10 mg once daily.

    – Carvedilol 3.125 mg twice daily increasing to with close monitoring 25–50 mg twice daily.

- Digoxin: improved symptoms, exercise capacity and fewer admissions to hospital.

- Nitrates and hydralazine: improved survival in symptomatic patients intolerant to ACE inhibitors or angiotensin II (AII) receptor antagonists.

- Amiodarone: prevention of arrhythmias in patients with *symptomatic* ventricular arrhythmias.

*Prefer long-acting drugs such as lisinopril or ramipril unless patient is haemodynamically unstable, in which case short-acting captopril once or twice daily is useful for initiating therapy

Table 5.1 Arrhythmias

Arrhythmia	Basic pathology	Medical management	Intervention or surgical management
Non-MI related			
AF or atrial flutter	Increasing prevalence with age	Control rate with digoxin/β blocker/amiodarone and restore to sinus rhythm by chemical (flecainide/amiodarone)/electrical cardioversion	Persistent flutter/fibrillation needs anticoagulation with warfarin and consideration for DC cardioversion, depending on underlying pathology. Electrophysiological ablation can be very successful and should be considered
	Look for possible underlying causes:	Heparin and/or warfarin needs to be considered	
	Cardiac: mitral valve disease, IHD, pericarditis, cardiomyopathy, endo-/myocarditis, post-cardiac surgery	If patient hypotensive consider immediate DC cardioversion	
	Atrial myxoma	Acute AF or flutter often reverts spontaneously within 24 h	Occasionally AV node ablation and a permanent pacemaker are needed to control heart rate for those not responsive to other medical therapy
	Lung pathology: pneumonia, pulmonary embolic malignancy, trauma/surgery	Correct underlying cause if possible	
	Metabolic: thyrotoxicosis, alcohol excess, electrolyte imbalance/acidosis		
SVT	Accessory pathway between atria and ventricles causing a re-entrant circuit, e.g. Wolff–Parkinson–White syndrome, AV node re-entrant tachycardia	DC cardioversion if hypotensive	Consider atrial overdrive pacing
		Vagal manoeuvres, e.g. carotid massage/Valsalva manoeuvre	Electrophysiology studies and ablation if medical treatment is not adequate
	Ectopic atrial focus or AF/atrial flutter	Intravenous adenosine (3–12 mg)	
		Consider intravenous verapamil or β blocker	
VT	Associated with IHD, hypertensive heart disease, cardiomyopathy	Synchronized DC cardioversion if hypotensive. If stable give intravenous lidocaine	Consider electrophysiological studies/ablation or implantable defibrillator
	Can be precipitated by bradycardia, hypokalaemia, hypomagnesaemia, MI or long Q–T interval	Correct metabolic abnormalities	
		Amiodarone may be necessary to stabilize patient	

Arrhythmia	Basic pathology	Medical management	Intervention or surgical management
Ventricular premature beats	Ectopic focus within ventricle	Treatment offers no benefit to survival Give anti-arrhythmic if symptomatic (β blocker)	
Torsades de pointes	Associated with inherited or acquired prolongation of Q–T interval, e.g. drugs, hypokalaemia, hypomagnesaemia, hypocalcaemia, IHD	Correct electrolyte imbalance Stop drugs prolonging Q–T interval Intravenous magnesium Consider β blocker in hereditary long Q–T interval	Consider temporary pacing
VF	See Case 5.4	See Case 5.4	See Case 5.4
Post-MI arrhythmias			
AF/flutter	AF is often transient post-MI	Rate control Usually reverts spontaneously Treat as above if persistent	
VF	Acute MI is a common cause of VF	As non-MI treatment Note that anti-arrhythmic drug treatment is not necessary after VF within the first 24 h of acute MI	Recurrent or late VF (> 48 h) indicates risk of subsequent sudden death and these patients should be considered for coronary angiography and electrophysiological studies
VT	Associated with IHD, especially acutely post-MI	Treatment as above Note that anti-arrhythmic drug treatment is not necessary after VT within the first 24 h of acute MI	Recurrent or late VT (> 48 h) indicates risk of subsequent sudden death and these patients should be considered for coronary angiography and electrophysiological studies
Ventricular premature beats	Common acutely post MI/post thrombolysis	Often no treatment is required	

Sinus bradycardia	Commonly complicates RV infarction/inferior infarction	If heart rate is < 60 beats/min with hypotension or cardiac failure, give atropine 0.6 mg i.v.	Temporary or permanent pacing may be needed
AV block	Commonly complicates RV infarction/inferior infarction	First-degree heart block requires no treatment. Second- and third-degree heart block with inferior infarction require treatment only if associated with hypotension, syncope, cardiac failure or 'escape' ventricular arrhythmias. Atropine 0.6 mg i.v. bolus up to 3 mg i.v. can be given	Temporary or permanent pacing may be needed Second- or third-degree heart block associated with anterior infarction should be always considered for temporary pacing because it may progress to ventricular standstill.

AF, atrial fibrillation; AV, atrioventricular; DC, direct current; IHD, ischaemic heart disease; MI, myocardial infarction; SVT, supraventricular tachycardia; VF, ventricular fibrillation; VT, ventricular tachycardia.

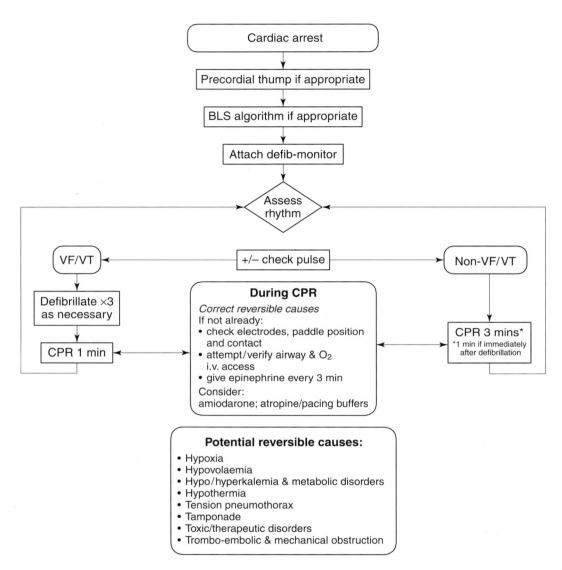

Figure 5.1 Universal ALS Algorithm

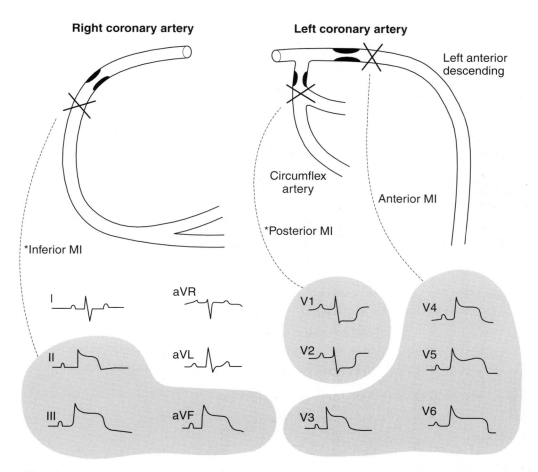

Right coronary artery

Left coronary artery

Left anterior
descending

Circumflex
artery

Anterior MI

*Posterior MI

*Inferior MI

I

aVR

II

aVL

V1

V4

III

aVF

V2

V5

V3

V6

*There is an overlap between inferior and posterior depending on the patient's anatomy, i.e. whether the RCA is the dominant artery or the circumflex.

Figure 5.2 Chest pain

Table 5.2 Valvular heart disease

	Cause	Symptoms	Signs	Management
Aortic stenosis	Degenerative (± calcification) Calcification of congenital bicuspid valve Occasionally rheumatic fever	Symptoms usually only occur when the aortic orifice is reduced to a third of its normal size: angina, dyspnoea and exercise-induced syncope	Slow rising pulse and narrow pulse pressure. Thrusting non-displaced or displaced apex. An ejection click may precede the harsh ejection systolic murmur which is loudest over the right upper sternal edge and radiates to the carotids	Valve replacement if symptomatic and high valve gradient on echocardiogram Valvuloplasty in young patients
Aortic regurgitation	Damage of aortic valve cusps: bicuspid aortic valve (congenital) infective endocarditis rheumatic fever Dilatation of aortic root/valve ring: arthritides, e.g. Reiter's syndrome, ankylosing spondylitis severe hypertension aortic dissection rare causes, e.g. Marfan's syndrome, syphilis	Usually asymptomatic unless severe. Exertional dyspnoea and fatigue	Collapsing pulse and wide pulse pressures. Nail-bed capillary pulsations (Quincke's sign), head nodding (deMusset's sign), and 'pistol shot' sounding femoral arteries are sometimes seen. Apex is laterally displaced and thrusting. There is an early diastolic murmur at the lower left sternal edge that is heard best with the patient sitting forward in full expiration	Diuretics and vasodilators for mild symptoms Valve replacement once patient is symptomatic or if the left ventricle is dilating

	Causes	Symptoms	Signs	Treatment
Mitral stenosis	Rheumatic fever	Exertional dyspnoea, cough ± haemoptysis, palpitations	AF, malar flush, palpable first heart sound ('tapping' apex). Loud first heart sound, opening snap in early diastole followed by rumbling mid-diastolic murmur at apex with presystolic accentuation. Pulmonary hypertension, RVH and eventually right heart failure	Valvuloplasty if valve is not calcified and no significant MR. Valve replacement
MR	Mitral valve prolapse (MVP) Rheumatic fever Papillary muscle dysfunction/rupture post-MI LV dilatation Endocarditis Rare causes: SLE, Marfan's syndrome	Exertional dyspnoea and lethargy. Pulmonary oedema if acute regurgitation	Laterally displaced apex. Soft first heart sound. Pansystolic murmur loudest at apex and radiating to axilla and throughout precordium. Third heart sound often present	Diuretics and ACE inhibitors. Valve repair or replacement if symptomatic or progressive LV dilatation
MVP	Unknown cause (more common in women) Associated with Marfan's syndrome/IHD	Usually asymptomatic. Can present with atypical chest pain or palpitations	Midsystolic click ± murmur. MR may occur	β Blockers if symptomatic
TS	Rheumatic fever Carcinoid	Usually associated with mitral and aortic valve disease which dominate the symptoms and signs		Valvuloplasty or valve replacement

	Cause	Symptoms	Signs	Management
TR	Raised pulmonary pressure (look for cause e.g. PE, lung disease, left heart causes [MV disease, LV dysfunction]) Can be physiological Rare causes: rheumatic heart disease, infective endocarditis, carcinoid	Symptoms and signs of underlying lung pathology may be present, and of right heart failure	Raised JVP with giant 'v' waves, pulsatile liver and pansystolic murmur at the lower left sternal edge, accentuated with inspiration. Peripheral oedema and ascites may be present	If functional, signs usually improve with diuretic therapy Annuloplasty or replacement very rarely required
PS	Congenital (usually with other defects, e.g. Fallot's tetralogy)	Fatigue, syncope, RV failure	Systolic murmur at the left sternal edge. Signs of right heart failure	Valvuloplasty Valve replacement
PR	Pulmonary hypertension Endocarditis (intravenous drug abusers)	Usually asymptomatic	Early diastolic murmur at the upper left sternal edge	Treatment rarely needed
VSD	Congenital Post-MI (ventricular septal rupture)	May be asymptomatic Eisenmenger's syndrome occurs later in life when pulmonary vascular disease develops	Pansystolic murmur loudest at the third or fourth intercostal space Pulmonary hypertension signs may be present	Repair of VSD
ASD	Congenital	Arrhythmias and heart failure	Wide fixed splitting of S2. Pulmonary ejection systolic murmur as a result of increased flow. Pulmonary hypertension with TR or PR may occur	Surgical or percutaneous closure if symptomatic or developing Eisenmenger's syndrome

ACE, angiotensin-converting enzyme; AR, aortic regurgitation; ASD, atrial septal defect; AF, atrial fibrillation; IHD, ischaemic heart disease; JVP, jugular venous pressure; LV, left ventricular; MI, myocardial infarction; MR, mitral regurgitation; MV, mitral valve; PE, pulmonary embolus; PR, pulmonary regurgitation; PS, pulmonary stenosis; RV, right ventricular; RVH, right ventricular hypertrophy; SLE, systemic lupus erythematosus; TR, tricuspid regurgitation; VSD, ventricular septal defect.

Answers

 CASE 5.1 – A 34-year-woman with palpitations.

 Q1: What specific questions would you ask the patient?

A1

Elicit from the history the onset of symptoms and any associated features (chest pain, dyspnoea, nausea, tremor, etc.). The patient's symptoms may be related to the arrhythmia or an ischaemic event might have caused it. The patient may be able to identify whether the rhythm is regular or irregular, or tap out the arrhythmia. Determine if the palpitations have occurred in the past. Ask specifically for precipitating or relieving factors, and for any medical conditions that the patient may have that predispose to arrhythmias, e.g. thyrotoxicosis, valvular heart disease. A drug history is very important because some drugs may precipitate arrhythmias or influence the arrhythmia's management (e.g. verapamil must not be given in patients already on β blockers because it may result in circulatory collapse).

 Q2: What is the most likely diagnosis?

A2

Atrial fibrillation (AF) secondary to thyrotoxicosis as a result of the history of diarrhoea and insomnia that are features in this condition. Other causes of arrhythmia to consider are described in the Key concepts.

Q3: What examination would you perform?

A3

A full physical examination is necessary. Determine the rate, character and volume of the pulse. Note if the patient is haemodynamically stable: record the blood pressure (BP) and examine for signs of heart failure. Auscultate for heart murmurs. Examine for thyroid status if appropriate.

 Q4: What would be the initial management?

A4

If the patient has a tachycardia and is haemodynamically unstable (systolic BP < 80 mmHg, reduced level of consciousness, severe pulmonary oedema) consider immediate DC (direct current) cardioversion. If the patient has a bradycardia and is haemodynamically compromised, give atropine 0.6–1.2 mg i.v. If there is persistent bradycardia, consider external pacing while organizing transvenous pacing wire insertion. See Key concepts.

Q5: What investigations would you request to confirm a diagnosis?

A5

Record a 12-lead ECG to determine the nature of the arrhythmia (regular versus irregular, narrow versus broad QRS complex). Take blood for routine haematology, biochemistry, calcium, magnesium, cardiac enzymes, thyroid function tests and glucose. A chest radiograph is useful to estimate heart size and look for signs of pulmonary oedema.

 Q6: What other issues should be addressed?

A6

This depends on the arrhythmia and its underlying cause (see Key concepts).

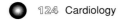 **CASE 5.2 – A 53-year-old man with sudden onset of chest pain.**

 Q1: What specific questions would you ask the patient?

A1

There is a wide range of differential diagnoses for chest pain and it is thus very important to establish the exact nature of the pain. A constricting central chest pain that occurs on exertion and is relieved by rest or GTN suggests angina. A similar crushing central chest pain when more prolonged and of greater severity indicates myocardial infarction (MI). Unlike angina this pain is not relieved by rest or GTN and is typically associated with extreme distress, sweating, nausea ± vomiting and dyspnoea. Cardiac pain usually radiates to one or both arms and up the neck to the jaw. Risk factors for IHD to seek are: diabetes mellitus, hypertension, hyperlipidaemia, smoking, and any family history of IHD. Male sex, increasing age and obesity are also risk factors. Other causes of chest pain to consider include: pericarditis, dissecting aortic aneurysm, pulmonary embolus (PE), pleurisy, gastro-oesophageal reflux, perforated peptic ulcer, pancreatitis and cholecystitis.

 Q2: What is the most likely diagnosis?

A2

The most likely diagnosis is MI. This is usually caused by rupture of an atherosclerotic plaque with formation of thrombus and complete occlusion of a coronary artery.

 Q3: What examination would you perform?

A3

A full physical examination is needed. The patient is usually very distressed and appears pale, grey and sweating. The pulse must be noted because arrhythmias are common, particularly if the MI is of the right coronary artery, which supplies the sinoatrial node. Hypotension may also occur and the BP is often measured in both arms to look for any significant difference (> 15 mmHg) that may indicate aortic dissection. The jugular venous pressure (JVP), if raised, indicates right heart failure and right ventricular (RV) infarction must be considered. Listen for any murmurs and then examine for pulmonary oedema. Cardiogenic shock can be recognized from the following: systolic BP < 90 mmHg, heart rate >100 beats/min or < 40 beats/min, the presence of pulmonary oedema (oxygen saturation < 90 per cent), cold peripheries, agitation or confusion and oliguria.

 Q4: What would be the initial management?

A4

Immediate treatment is aimed at relief of pain, limitation of infarct size and management of complications if they arise. Oxygen is administered via a facemask (28 per cent if history of chronic bronchitis/emphysema) and the patient is attached to an ECG monitor. Intravenous access is obtained and 5 mg diamorphine given along with 10 mg metoclopramide as an antiemetic. Further 2.5 mg boluses of diamorphine should be given until the patient is pain free. Soluble aspirin 300 mg and sublingual GTN (provided that the patient is not hypotensive) must also be given if not already administered by the ambulance paramedics. A 12-lead ECG is done as a priority to decide whether thrombolysis is appropriate. Thrombolysis given within 4 h of pain onset, using streptokinase or recombinant tissue plasminogen activator (rtPA) with intravenous heparin, will achieve reperfusion in 50–70 per cent of patients (compared with 20 per cent of controls). Primary coronary angioplasty should be considered if available. See Key concepts.

 Q5: What investigations would you request to confirm a diagnosis?

A5

The diagnosis is usually made on the basis of a history and 12-lead ECG, and confirmed later with a rise in cardiac enzymes. ST-segment elevation on the ECG occurs within minutes and is followed by T-wave inversion that persists after the ST segment returns to baseline. The indication of transmural infarction is the development of Q waves, usually hours or days later. The infarct site may be determined by the location of ECG changes. Other ischaemic changes on the ECG that may occur are new left bundle-branch block (LBBB), right bundle-branch block (RBBB), tachy- or bradyarrhythmias, left or right axis deviation or atrioventricular (AV) block. Creatine phosphokinase (CPK) is the cardiac enzyme routinely measured (rises at 4–8 h, peaks at 24 h and returns to normal in 3–4 days) but the CK-MB isoenzyme and troponin myofibrillar protein (rises within 4 h and remains elevated for up to 2 weeks) are more specific for myocardial disease and diagnostically more reliable. A chest radiograph to determine cardiac size and look for pulmonary oedema must be performed. Blood must be taken for routine haematology and biochemistry investigations, and for random glucose and cholesterol measurement.

 Q6: What other issues should be addressed?

A6

Patients should be admitted to the coronary care unit (CCU) if possible and have bedrest for 24–36 h. Subcutaneous heparin is used as prophylaxis against deep venous thrombosis (DVT). Uncomplicated MI patients can be discharged home after 5 days. Complications that may occur include: cardiogenic shock, reinfarction, dysrhythmias, pericarditis, acute mitral regurgitation (AMR), ventricular septal defect (VSD) and myocardial rupture. In cases where pain persists or there is no resolution of ST elevation, patients are considered for repeat thrombolysis or referred for urgent angiography with the aim of revascularization, usually by coronary angioplasty. Secondary prevention post-MI is important and each patient will be prescribed aspirin, a β-adrenoceptor blocker, ACE inhibitor and a lipid-lowering statin, unless specific contraindications are present. On discharge, patients should be advised to inform the DVLA (Driver and Vehicle Licensing Authority) of their admission; they can usually resume driving in 6 weeks and return to work in 3 months. Every patient should be entered into a cardiac rehabilitation programme and have active follow-up.

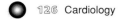 **CASE 5.3 – An 80-year-old patient collapses, requiring CPR.**

 Q1: What specific questions would you ask the patient?

A1

Obtain as much history as possible from the daughter and paramedics. Events immediately preceding the arrest are particularly important because they may indicate the cause. Enquire specifically about any illness that the patient may have had and obtain a past medical history: IHD, diabetes mellitus (consider hypoglycaemia), depression (drug overdoses), etc. Establish the medication that she is on and enquire about illicit drug use if appropriate (especially in a young patient where examination may yield evidence of intravenous drug abuse). It is also important to identify the length of time before resuscitation and the duration of resuscitation before admission. Without CPR, permanent cerebral dysfunction occurs after 3–4 min of cardiopulmonary arrest. The longer the period of arrest, the less likely it is that resuscitation will be successful and the patient restored to a healthy life.

 Q2: What is the most likely diagnosis?

A2

The most common cause of a cardiac arrest is ventricular fibrillation (VF). Other causes include other dysrhythmias (pulseless ventricular tachycardia, brady-dysrhythmia), sudden pump failure (MI), circulatory obstruction (PE) and cardiovascular rupture (myocardial rupture/dissecting aortic aneurysm).

 Q3: What examination would you perform?

A3

The initial assessment of the airway/breathing/circulation (ABC) would have already been performed by the paramedics. Examine the patient briefly to check that CPR is effective: palpate for a pulse and check that both lungs are ventilated. Look for any signs of bleeding such as haematemesis or melaena that may suggest hypovolaemia as the cause of the arrest. If the abdomen is distended, an intra-abdominal catastrophe such as a ruptured abdominal aortic aneurysm may be suspected.

 Q4: What would be the initial management?

A4

Effective basic life support (BLS) and early defibrillation are the most vital elements of successful resuscitation. The patient is already being resuscitated by the paramedics and intravenous access has usually been established. Attach the patient to a defibrillator via ECG leads to determine whether the cardiac rhythm is 'shockable' (VF/pulseless ventricular tachycardia [VT]) or not (asystole/electromechanical dissociation). If the patient is in a 'shockable' rhythm, DC cardioversion should be given without delay. Continue advanced CPR according to the algorithm determined by the patient's cardiac rhythm each time it is assessed (see Key concepts). The patient should be intubated if this has not already been done. Adrenaline or epinephrine (1 mg i.v.) should be given every 3 min and, if the patient is in asystole, 3 mg atropine should be given once only. In refractory VF/VT (after four cycles of advanced life support [ALS]), amiodarone is recommended. An arterial blood gas is taken during ALS and if hyperkalaemia is present, calcium chloride is administered. Bicarbonate can be given in severe acidosis (pH<7.0) and in hyperkalaemia. Treatable causes must be considered (see algorithm) and where possible an attempt at correcting them made.

 Q5: What investigations would you request to confirm a diagnosis?

A5

In the event of successful resuscitation a 12-lead ECG must be done to look for evidence of MI that may have precipitated the arrest. A chest radiograph may show pulmonary oedema or identify rib fractures secondary to vigorous CPR, and is useful to check the position of the endotracheal (ET) tube. Routine blood biochemistry, haematology, cardiac enzymes, glucose, and group and save are taken, and blood cross-matched if a bleed is suspected. An arterial blood gas (ABG) will indicate whether ventilation is adequate.

 Q6: What other issues should be addressed?

A6

Most patients need admission to intensive care post-arrest and may require ventilation and support with inotropes such as adrenaline. They may require a central line. A member of the medical team must speak with the family and inform them of the future management and likely prognosis.

● **CASE 5.4 – A 65-year-old with tearing chest pain.**

  Q1: What specific questions would you ask the patient?

A1

Establish the nature of the pain. Aortic dissection pain can mimic MI, and caution must be taken to distinguish the two because treatment is different. Abrupt onset of tearing chest pain that radiates to the back and abdomen indicates dissection. Patients may present with symptoms and signs of occlusion of one or more of the branches of the aorta as the dissection progresses: stroke, limb ischaemia, paraplegia, MI. Risk factors to enquire about include: hypertension, arteriosclerosis (IHD/peripheral vascular disease [PVD]), pregnancy or a history of trauma, and rarely Marfan's syndrome.

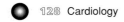 **Q2: What is the most likely diagnosis?**

A2

The most likely diagnosis is aortic dissection. This may be proximal (type I starts in ascending aorta but progress down the aorta, type II is localized to ascending aorta) or distal (type III starts in the descending aorta after the arch), involving the descending aorta only.

 Q3: What examination would you perform?

A3

A full examination is necessary. A BP difference between the right and the left arm (> 15 mmHg) occurs in 10 per cent of patients with a dissection. A difference in pulse between right and left arm or radial to femoral pulse. An elevated JVP and pulsus paradox indicate cardiac tamponade caused by rupture of the aortic wall into the pericardium. Aortic regurgitation may be heard when the aortic root is involved. Examine for any neurological deficit.

 Q4: What would be the initial management?

A4

Resuscitation is the initial management. Oxygen must be given via a facemask. Intravenous access is established and pain relief with diamorphine given. Systolic BP must be reduced to 100–120 mmHg using drugs that decrease the inotropic force of the heart, e.g. labetolol infusion.

 Q5: What investigations would you request to confirm a diagnosis?

A5

The diagnosis of aortic dissection can be made in several ways. The diagnosis is often suspected from the chest radiograph, which may demonstrate a widened mediastinum. However, this is an unreliable sign and chest computed tomography (CT) with contrast or magnetic resonance imaging (MRI) is usually preferred to make the diagnosis non-invasively. An echocardiogram is also useful to look at the aortic root in detail in type I or II dissection, but a transoesophageal echocardiogram is preferred if possible to obtain detailed views of the descending thoracic aorta. Cardiac catheterization will aid planning of surgical repair.

 Q6: What other issues should be addressed?

A6

Over 50 per cent of patients die in the first 24 h of presentation. Urgent surgical repair is needed in type I or II dissection, and frequently in type III, if the patient is to have a chance of survival.

CASE 5.5 – A 25-year-old man with a heart murmur.

 Q1: What specific questions would you ask the patient?

A1

Elicit from the history whether the patient has any symptoms suggestive of valvular stenosis or regurgitation: dyspnoea, oedema, dizziness, syncope, palpitations or chest pain. Haemoptysis or recurrent bronchitis may indicate pulmonary hypertension. A past medical history may suggest a cause, e.g. rheumatic heart disease, MI causing papillary muscle rupture. Consider underlying conditions and family history that may predispose to valvular abnormalities, e.g. dilated or hypertrophic cardiomyopathy, Marfan's syndrome or ankylosing spondylitis. Ask about any symptoms that may suggest endocarditis (rash, fevers) or predisposing factors such as intravenous drug abuse.

 Q2: What is the most likely diagnosis?

A2

A heart murmur is heard when there is turbulent blood flow, the cause usually being an abnormal heart valve that may be incompetent (regurgitant), stenotic or both. An 'innocent murmur' produced by a normal heart valve tends to occur in the setting of a hyperdynamic circulation, e.g. anaemia, thyrotoxicosis, pregnancy. See Key concepts for causes of each murmur.

 Q3: What examination would you perform?

A3

A full physical examination is necessary. Determine the characteristics of the pulse and BP. Look for signs of right heart failure: raised JVP, ankle oedema, enlarged liver and for pulmonary oedema indicating LV failure. Determine whether the murmur is systolic or diastolic. The character of the murmur (e.g. pansystolic in mitral regurgitation) and the location and radiation of the murmur will give further clues to the diagnosis (see Key concepts). Bear in mind that a soft, midsystolic murmur that varies with posture and is not associated with signs of heart disease is usually benign.

Q4: What would be the initial management?

A4

Medical therapy is mainly aimed at treatment of complications (AF, heart failure). Surgical treatment may be valve repair, valve replacement or valvotomy (see Key concepts). Surgery must be performed before irreversible LV dysfunction and pulmonary oedema become established.

Q5: What investigations would you request to confirm a diagnosis?

A5

Valve dysfunction is confirmed with echocardiography ± cardiac catheterization (to define the haemodynamics of the lesion). An ECG may show LV hypertrophy and confirm AF or, if in sinus rhythm, show the bifid P wave ('P mitrale') of left atrial hypertrophy in mitral stenosis or the tall P wave ('P pulmonale') of pulmonary hypertension. A chest radiograph may indicate cardiomegaly.

Q6: What other issues should be addressed?

A6

Prosthetic valves are either mechanical (e.g. Starr–Edwards ball-and-cage valve, Björk–Shiley tilting disc valve) or bioprosthetic valves (porcine xenograft). Bioprosthetic pig valves typically degenerate after about 10 years and are hence preferably used in elderly people. Mechanical valves last longer but need lifelong anticoagulation. All prosthetic valves and native abnormal valves are susceptible to infection. Patients should always be advised that antibiotic prophylaxis is necessary if they undergo any procedure that may induce bacteraemia, e.g. surgical or dental procedures.

⚇ OSCE Counselling Cases – Answers

OSCE COUNSELLING CASE 5.1 – 'Can I stop my warfarin (anticoagulation in a patient with prosthetic heart valve)?'

The answer is definitely NO! Anticoagulation must never be stopped in a patient with a metal heart valve.

If she stops anticoagulation, there is a significant risk of thrombosis, especially in the hypercoagulable state of pregnancy. A clot may obstruct the valve, causing sudden stenosis, or embolize and cause a stroke.

However, her worries are genuine. Warfarin does indeed have teratogenic effects and can also cause intracerebral haemorrhage in the fetus. Women that continue warfarin throughout pregnancy have approximately a 7 per cent chance of having a baby with a congenital abnormality and a further 16 per cent risk of stillbirth or spontaneous abortion. There are also increased complications after delivery.

The answer is to advise the patient to change to heparin for the first 3 months of the pregnancy, restart warfarin at 3 months and change again to heparin 2–4 weeks before the expected delivery date. Heparin is not teratogenic but it must be noted that it is also associated with a higher risk of abortion and a higher incidence of bleeding.

Another point of note is that warfarin is excreted in breast milk (in small amounts) and it is advisable that mothers on warfarin should not breast-feed if possible.

OSCE COUNSELLING CASE 5.2 – The use of anti-anginal medication.

GTN

Nitrates are potent vasodilators, but the main benefit in angina is by causing a reduction in venous return, which reduces LV work. Sublingual GTN is used to treat symptoms in angina on an as-required basis. It comes in spray or tablet form, with the advantage of the spray having longer storage life once opened. The onset of action is 1–2 min and effects last for up to 20 min. Sublingual GTN can be taken repeatedly but patients should be advised to seek medical attention if they do not get any relief after repeated use.

Headaches are common, especially in the first few days after starting treatment. Patients can be advised that if the headache is severe they can spit the tablet out or swallow it in order to deactivate it. Flushing and postural hypotension causing syncopal attacks are also reported and may limit therapy.

β BLOCKERS

β Blockers decrease myocardial oxygen demand by causing a fall in heart rate, BP and decreasing myocardial contractility. However, they are contraindicated in asthma and chronic obstructive pulmonary disease (COPD), and relatively contraindicated in diabetes mellitus, PVD and severe LV dysfunction.

Lethargy is a common side effect and interference with exercise capacity may cause patients to discontinue their medication. Coldness of extremities and sleep disturbances may also lead to non-compliance. Bradycardia and other conduction disorders may also occur.

OSCE COUNSELLING CASE 5.3 – 'I have heart failure. Do I need to take my medications for life?'

Unfortunately a diagnosis of heart failure (in this case moderate to severe on echocardiogram) is associated with a worse prognosis than most cancers (50 per cent 5-year mortality rate if untreated). With correct therapeutic management his symptoms will improve and his annual risk of death will be cut by half.

It is very important to use medications that have been used in large randomized trials that have been shown to be effective (see Key concepts).

Ask the patient whether he is having any particular problem with the drugs prescribed, particularly symptoms of hypotension.

Advise the patient that, if possible, the dose of bisoprolol may be increased to try to get to the target dose of 10 mg once daily.

Advise the patient that he will require regular blood checks (initially 1–2 weekly and then 3 monthly watching for hyperkalaemia and rising creatinine) because of the potential interaction between ACE inhibitors and spironolactone.

In addition the patient should be advised to monitor his weight regularly and seek advice should it rise because it may be a sign of fluid overload.

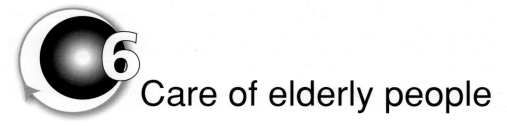

6 Care of elderly people

Peter Wallis

FALLS

Q1: What is the differential diagnosis?
Q2: What features in the history support the diagnosis?
Q3: What additional features in the history would you seek to support the potential diagnoses?
Q4: What other features would you look for on clinical examination?
Q5: What investigations would you perform?
Q6: What treatment options are available?

Clinical cases

CASE 6.1 – A 71-year-old man has been brought to the accident and emergency department (A&E) after a fall whilst shopping.

He lost consciousness momentarily and has little recollection of the event. He admits to previous episodes of dizziness, sometimes on exertion and often associated with shortness of breath.

His past history includes a hiatus hernia, diverticular disease, and osteoarthritis of his neck and knees. He is taking regular omeprazole, a dietary fibre supplement and a compound analgesic containing paracetamol and codeine (codamol).

Examination discloses a regular pulse and blood pressure (BP) of 114/76 mmHg. There is an ejection systolic cardiac murmur radiating to the neck. The lung fields are clear. Neurological examination is normal.

CASE 6.2 – An 82-year-old woman presents with recurrent falls.

She is housebound. Her most recent fall occurred while getting up to go to the toilet at night. She has arthritis, heart failure and poor vision as a result of macular degeneration, and has had a previous hip replacement. She receives treatment with furosemide, ramipril, co-codamol (paracetamol/codeine compound analgesic), dothiepin and temazepam.

She is very frail. The main findings on examination are: abbreviated mental test 6/10, vision – large print only, kyphotic spine, brisk reflexes bilaterally; peripheral oedema, clear lung fields and normal jugular venous pressure (JVP); heart rate (HR) 112/min atrial fibrillation (AF); BP sitting 114/62 mmHg, mitral regurgitation.

CASE 6.3 – A 78-year-old man who lives alone is brought to A&E after being found on the floor at home by his neighbour.

He is confused and disorientated. His head is bruised and he appears unkempt. He is immobile and there is cog-wheel rigidity in all his limbs. There are no focal neurological signs. Reflexes are hard to elicit as a result of the muscle stiffness. Plantar responses are down-going. There are signs of a lower respiratory tract infection. Temperature is 38.2°C, BP 102/60 mmHg, HR 94/min.

Investigation discloses:

- Normal plasma glucose and electrolytes

- Urea 24 mmol/L

- Creatinine 142 μmol/L

- Haemoglobin (Hb) 15.5 g/dL

- White cell count (WCC) 14.3 × 10^9/L

- Platelets 342 × 10^9/L

- Chest radiograph: consolidation right lower lobe

- ECG: sinus tachycardia.

👥 OSCE Counselling Cases

OSCE COUNSELLING CASE 6.1 – What advice would you give?

An elderly housebound woman has fallen at home on several occasions and has recently attended A&E with a Colles' (wrist) fracture. Her daughter is concerned about the presence of osteoporosis and seeks your advice at the surgery about the need for calcium tablets in order to prevent further fractures.

OSCE COUNSELLING CASE 6.2 – A house-bound 94-year-old woman with epilepsy (controlled with phenytoin) presents with falls, weakness and generalized aches and pains.

Biochemical tests reveal:

- Calcium (corrected) 1.85 mmol/L (normal range 2.05–2.60 mmol/L)

- Phosphate 0.68 mmol/L (normal range 0.8–1.45 mmol/L)

- Albumin 32 g/L (normal range 35–48 g/L)

- Alkaline phosphatase (ALP) 458 U/L (normal range 30–200 U/L).

Q1: What is the likely diagnosis?

Q2: What factors might have precipitated this condition?

Q3: What signs would you look for on examination?

Q4: How would you treat the condition?

🔑 Key concepts

In order to work through the core clinical cases in this chapter, you will need to understand the following key concepts.

Older people are at much greater risk of falling and most falls occur at home. Nevertheless the risk of falling is much higher in those older people who reside in an institutional environment such as a residential or nursing home or hospital, as a result of the increased frailty of this group. One-third of people aged over 65 will fall in a year, often repeatedly. Falls resulting in injury are a leading cause of death in older people, accounting for two-thirds of injury-related deaths in those aged 85 and over. Of course, most falls do not result in death, but can give rise to substantial morbidity. The fear of falling often leads to loss of confidence, increased dependence on others and restriction of activity.

Most patients fall because of age-related and/or disease-associated damage to one or more systems essential for the maintenance of balance and posture. Vision, vestibular, sensory, locomotor, cardiovascular and central processing mechanisms are all important in this regard. A careful history detailing the circumstances surrounding the fall is essential. Often there is little recollection of the prodromal events, so corroborative information from a witness is invaluable. Accurate diagnosis, treatment of predisposing illness and amelioration of risk factors such as impaired vision, polypharmacy, inadequate footwear and environmental hazards are all important. Multidisciplinary falls clinics (with physiotherapy and occupational therapy support) and exercise programmes can reduce the risk of falling.

Many falls result in bone fractures. Effective treatments for osteoporosis in older patients include bisphosphonates as well as calcium and vitamin D supplements. The latter are preferred for older people who are housebound or cared for in a residential or nursing home setting. Hip protectors can reduce the risk of femoral neck fractures in selected frail older people when worn.

Answers

 CASE 6.1 – A 71-year-old man has been brought to A&E after a fall whilst shopping.

 Q1: What is the differential diagnosis?

A1

- Aortic stenosis
- Cardiac arrhythmia
- Silent myocardial infarction (MI)
- Postural hypotension
- Vasovagal episode
- Vertebrobasilar transient ischaemic attack (TIA).

 Q2: What features in the history support the diagnosis?

A2

The syncopal event occurred on exertion and this is consistent with significant aortic stenosis. In this situation, syncope can be precipitated by impaired cardiac output or a transient arrhythmia such as ventricular tachycardia. The history of previous exertional dizziness and breathlessness lends support to this diagnosis.

Silent MI and/or cardiac arrhythmia must be considered too. Myocardial infarction can present without chest pain, particularly in older patients.

Postural hypotension – postural dizziness when standing (e.g. arising from bed at night) – might be volunteered. Enquire about medications with hypotensive properties (e.g. diuretics, antihypertensives, antidepressants). Co-proxamol is not usually a cause of postural hypotension, but the opiate component (dextropropoxyphene) can impair balance.

Vasovagal episodes are a common cause of syncopal events, particularly in younger patients. In this case, the presence of other cardiac symptoms and signs makes the diagnosis unlikely.

Finally, the patient does have an arthritic neck. When severe, this can compromise the vertebrobasilar circulation, especially if there is significant atheroma affecting the vertebrobasilar system and circle of Willis. The apparent absence of sudden neck movement before syncope and the lack of other features such as dizziness, vertigo or sudden loss of tone in the legs ('drop attack') makes this diagnosis less likely.

 Q3: What additional features in the history would you seek to support the potential diagnoses?

A3

The presence of exertional chest pain (angina) and dyspnoea supports the diagnosis of aortic stenosis (SAD = syncope, angina, dyspnoea).

Q4: What other features would you look for on clinical examination?

A4

Aortic stenosis – the following might be present:

- Ejection systolic murmur radiating to the neck
- Slow rising pulse
- Low pulse pressure
- Ejection click sometimes heard
- Early diastolic murmur if there is also aortic regurgitation
- Quiet second heart sound

Silent MI

- Signs of heart failure
- Cool, clammy peripheries resulting from low cardiac output

Postural hypotension

- Fall in standing BP < 20 mmHg associated with symptoms of dizziness/faintness

Vertebroasilar ischaemia.

- Symptoms are sometimes precipitated by head movement.

Q5: What investigations would you perform?

A5

ECG, chest radiograph, cardiac enzymes and/or troponin testing, echocardiography and ECG (Holter) monitoring. Full blood count, uka and electrolytes and blood glucose also necessary.

Q6: What treatment options are available?

A6

- A precise diagnosis is essential first. If aortic stenosis is severe, referral to a cardiologist for consideration of valve replacement. The patient should be advised to avoid sudden strenuous exertion in the meantime.
- Admission necessary if MI or arrhythmia suspected.
- Postural hypotension: discontinuation or reduced dose of offending medication, avoidance of precipitating events, compression hosiery.
- Aspirin for TIA.

CASE 6.2 – An 82-year-old woman presents with recurrent falls.

 Q1: What is the differential diagnosis?

A1

Multiple causes including:

- Poor vision
- Postural hypotension
- Polypharmacy
- Neurological dysfunction: previous strokes, cervical myelopathy, vitamin B_{12} deficiency all possible
- Arthritis/Osteomalacia
- Arrhythmia – atrial fibrillation (AF).

 Q2: What features in the history support the diagnosis?

A2

- Poor vision: the fall occurred at night when environmental hazards are more difficult to see and avoid.
- Postural hypotension: the fall occurred while getting out of bed to go to the toilet. She is on a lot of medications that can impair postural BP control, i.e. a diuretic, an angiotensin-converting enzyme (ACE) inhibitor and dothiepin (a tricyclic antidepressant with anticholinergic properties).
- Polypharmacy: postural hypotension as above:
  - impaired balance and cognition caused by temazepam, opiate analgesic and tricyclic antidepressant
  - muscle weakness: diuretic-induced hypokalaemia.
- Neurological dysfunction: brisk reflexes are suggestive of upper motor neuron (UMN) dysfunction. Common causes at this age include stroke disease, cervical myelopathy and occasionally vitamin B_{12} deficiency. As a result of the history of falls, a chronic subdural haematoma should be considered as well.
- AF: poorly controlled (rapid) ventricular rate on exertion causing syncope. AF might also be a manifestation of sick sinus syndrome, predisposing to supraventricular tachycardia or bradycardia.

 Q3: What additional features in the history would you seek to support the potential diagnoses?

A3

- Poor vision: access to spectacles, ability to read or identify objects, adequacy of lighting in the home.
- Postural hypotension: dizziness or falls when upright with associated symptoms of faintness or even syncope with rapid recovery when recumbent.

● Polypharmacy: concordance with medication regimen and any potential to exceed the intended dosing schedule.

● Neurological dysfunction.

● History suggestive of previous stroke or TIA.

● Neck arthritis with giddiness on head movement (especially looking upwards), pain radiating to shoulders/upper limbs (cervical spondylitic radiculopathy) would both suggest cervical myelopathy as a potential cause of falling.

● Enquire about diet, previous gastric surgery, bowel (terminal ileal) resection, anaemia and symptoms of sensory neuropathy in suspected vitamin B_{12} deficiency.

● Fluctuating alertness (and confusion) or consciousness with history of falls and head injuries (even trivial) should highlight the possibility of subdural intracranial bleeding.

● Bone pains and muscle weakness in a housebound woman with poor diet point to osteomalacia.

● Cardiac arrhythmia: recurrent episodes of dizziness and/or syncope unrelated to posture or activity with prompt recovery suggests an intermittent cardiac rhythm disturbance.

Q4: What other features would you look for on clinical examination?

A4

● Poor vision: Snellen chart to assess visual acuity, examination of eyes for common causes of visual loss in elderly people, i.e. refractive disorder, cataracts, glaucoma, macular degeneration.

● Postural hypotension: lying and standing BP.

● Neurological disorders: thorough central nervous system (CNS) examination essential. Focal UMN signs suggestive of stroke or subdural haematoma. Upgoing plantar responses, consistent with cervical myelopathy; peripheral neuropathy and posterior column dysfunction (joint position/vibration sense), suggest vitamin B_{12} deficiency.

● Arthritis/osteomalacia: joint examination, back pain, muscle weakness.

Q5: What investigations would you perform?

A5

The following tests are necessary:

● Lying and standing BP

● ECG

● Plasma urea and electrolytes (U&Es) and glucose

● Full blood count (FBC) (and vitamin B_{12}/folate levels if macrocytic anaemia present)

● Radiograph of painful bones/significantly arthritic joints

● Calcium, albumin and ALP (osteomalacia).

● Thyroid function tests

Other tests might be indicated after preliminary assessment and investigation:

- Cervical spine radiograph
- Computed tomography (CT) of the brain.

 Q6: What treatment options are available?

A6

- Vision: occupational therapist home visit to remove environmental hazards and improve lighting, assess for spectacles, ophthalmic referral as needed.
- Postural hypotension/polypharmacy: review need for and doses of all medications.
- Neurological dysfunction: B$_{12}$ replacement if deficiency, consider neurosurgical intervention if indicated (subdural haematoma, cervical myelopathy).
- Osteomalacia: calcium and vitamin D supplements.
- AF: digoxin/amiodarone, etc. Bradyarrhythmia will require assessment for cardiac pacemaker.

⬤ **CASE 6.3 – A 78-year-old man who lives alone is brought to A&E after being found on the floor at home by his neighbour.**

 Q1: What is the differential diagnosis?

A1

- Pneumonia
- Dehydration
- Parkinsonism
- Head injury with intracranial bleed or contusion.

 Q2: What features in the history support the diagnosis?

A2

Hypostatic pneumonia and dehydration often complicate a long period of immobility after a fall. Aspiration pneumonia should also be considered.

Parkinsonism: the generalized muscle 'cog-wheel' rigidity is suggestive of parkinsonism. Reflexes can be difficult to elicit in this situation. Spasticity caused by cerebrovascular disease would more usually be associated with hyperreflexia and upgoing plantar responses. Parkinsonism might be a result of idiopathic Parkinson's disease or secondary to other causes such as medication (e.g. neuroleptics – haloperidol, risperidone, etc.). His unkempt state suggests a chronic insidious decline before this acute presentation. Parkinson's disease could present in this way.

Head injury is obvious on examination, but the severity is difficult to assess. A subdural haematoma (acute and/or chronic) must be considered in this setting.

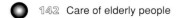

Q3:   What additional features in the history would you seek to support the potential diagnoses?

A3

Further history from family or neighbours, etc. is essential to establish the time course and pattern of his decline, as well as any history of previous falls. An accurate medication history is required, from the GP's records if necessary. Any suggestion of alcohol abuse is important.

Q4:   What other features would you look for on clinical examination?

A4

Assessment of conscious level and airway is essential because he is at risk of airway obstruction and aspiration.

Signs of weight loss and/or lymphadenopathy (tuberculosis [TB]) as well as clubbing (bronchial carcinoma).

The rigidity of parkinsonism is usually of 'lead-pipe' or 'cog-wheel' type. A 'pill-rolling', resting tremor might also be present.

Search for evidence of urinary outflow obstruction (enlarged bladder), faecal impaction (per rectum examination), bony injuries (hip, skull) and pressure sores, which can be overlooked in this setting.

Q5:   What investigations would you perform?

A5

Additional investigations:

- Arterial oxygen saturation/blood gases
- Blood and sputum cultures: pneumonia
- Calcium: confusion caused by hypercalcaemia
- ECG: arrhythmia
- Radiographs of skull and sites of other apparent bony injuries
- CT of head: acute or chronic subdural haematoma.

Q6:   What treatment options are available?

A6

- Rehydration with monitoring of urine output

- Oxygen therapy as directed by O_2 saturation and/or arterial blood gas (ABG) measurements
- Broad-spectrum antibiotics for hypostatic/aspiration pneumonia (e.g. benzylpenicillin, levofloxacin and metronidazole)
- Discontinuation of any drugs likely to cause parkinsonism
- If idiopathic Parkinson's disease is suspected, gradual introduction of L-dopa-based medication once resuscitation completed.

👥 OSCE Counselling Cases – Answers

OSCE COUNSELLING CASE 6.1 – What advice would you give?

The daughter has a valid point, but you will need to explain that to prevent further fractures measures are needed to reduce the risk of falling as well as a consideration of treatment for osteoporosis.

The patient would benefit from a multidisciplinary assessment in order to identify remediable medical illnesses that might precipitate falls (e.g. cardiovascular disease, medications, poor eyesight, Parkinson's disease). Advice from a physiotherapist or occupational therapist on measures to enhance fitness and safety at home and to secure help if further falls supervene, is also essential.

Osteoporosis can be assumed in this setting as a result of the presence of a low trauma fracture. Having excluded secondary causes of osteoporosis (e.g. thyrotoxicosis, steroid therapy, multiple myeloma, hyperparathyroidism), treatment for age-associated osteoporosis should be considered. In this setting calcium and vitamin D supplements are helpful and relatively safe, although it is prudent to measure the plasma calcium level before and 6–8 weeks after initiating treatment. A regular bisphosphonate is more controversial. The requirements for safe and effective oral dosing are somewhat cumbersome and restricting and should be discussed carefully with the patient before initiating treatment.

OSCE COUNSELLING CASE 6.2 – A house-bound 94-year-old woman with epilepsy (controlled with phenytoin) presents with falls, weakness and generalized aches and pains.

A1

Osteomalacia.

A2

Lack of exposure to sunlight, poor diet if socially isolated and/or poor health, impaired metabolism of vitamin D as a result of treatment with phenytoin (an enzyme inducer). Diseases causing malabsorption and chronic renal failure can also predispose to osteomalacia.

A3

Proximal muscle weakness, bony tenderness (pseudofractures or Looser's zones on radiograph), skeletal deformity such as kyphosis and bowing of limbs. Significant hypocalcaemia can precipitate tetany with a positive Chvostek sign (spasm of the facial muscles on tapping over the branches of the facial nerve in front of the ear) and Trousseau's sign (spasm of the hand and forearm muscles after compression of the forearm).

A4

Check blood level for 25-hydroxy-vitamin D and give vitamin D supplements either orally or intramuscularly. An adequate calcium intake should also be provided, if necessary with oral calcium supplements (1 g/day).

IMMOBILITY

Clinical cases

● **CASE 6.4 – A 74-year-old man who has difficulty walking is referred to the elderly medicine day hospital.**

He is confined to his chair unless assisted to stand. He cannot get into bed at night. His past history includes neck surgery for cervical spondylosis. He has hypertension treated with nifedipine.

He is obese, his legs are oedematous and he is incontinent of urine. He has ulceration and cellulitis affecting his lower legs. CNS examination reveals normal cognition and cranial nerves, but weak arms and legs (power 4/5), brisk reflexes bilaterally and upgoing plantar responses. His feet are warm but foot pulses are impossible to assess as a result of oedema.

● **CASE 6.5 – You have been called to see a 72-year-old man who lives alone at home.**

The district nurse has become increasingly concerned about his health. The patient has been house-bound for some time, but is now unable to rise from his chair. He is a large man and his left hip is very painful. There is no history of a fall. He is unkempt and his clothes smell of urine. He is a heavy smoker, and is breathless and wheezy with a chronic cough. His legs are swollen and blistered. Detailed examination is difficult, but does reveal signs of airflow obstruction, cyanosis, elevated JVP and peripheral oedema. Movement at the left hip is restricted and painful.

He is very reluctant to leave his home.

● **CASE 6.6 – A 68-year-old, previously active, woman is now unable to walk or stand having sustained a stroke (right middle cerebral artery territory infarction) 3 weeks previously.**

She has a dense left hemiparesis, homonymous hemianopia and sensory disturbance. She is also dysphasic and has difficulty swallowing. Recovery has been complicated by aspiration pneumonia. She has a urinary catheter and needs regular toileting. She is in AF, BP 142/78 mmHg. She is reluctant to engage with her programme of rehabilitation.

👥 OSCE Counselling Cases

OSCE COUNSELLING CASE 6.3 – A 75-year-old man who lives in a nursing home is confined to his bed or chair as a result of a previous left-sided stroke.

He is a large man and his care is made even more challenging as a result of the presence of dysphasia, dysphagia and mild cognitive impairment. The patient's GP periodically visits the nursing home to review his care and general condition.

List five important areas that the GP should enquire about or assess when visiting. Give a brief explanation as to why each of these areas needs review.

OSCE COUNSELLING CASE 6.4 – A 65-year-old woman is reviewed in clinic following recent colonic surgery.

Shortly after surgery she developed a hot swollen leg from a deep vein thrombosis (DVT), confirmed on duplex scanning. She has been started on anticoagulation therapy.

She is upset that this developed and wants to you to explain why it occurred and what was done to prevent it.

How would you approach answering this woman?

OSCE COUNSELLING CASE 6.5 – The wife of an elderly man is distressed because her husband's attendance at the local elderly care day hospital for physiotherapy has been discontinued.

He unfortunately suffered a severe stroke 3 months ago and is now confined to a wheelchair. He has difficulty speaking as a result of dysphasia.

What advice should be given?

🔑 Key concepts

In order to work through the core clinical cases in this chapter, you will need to understand the following key concepts.

Many chronic diseases in older people present with difficulty walking or even transferring from chair to bed, etc. Immobility itself is, of course, not a diagnosis but a symptom for which there might be any number of causes. Common illnesses in older people, which impair walking, include:

- Stroke disease
- Osteoarthritis
- Parkinsonism
- Dementia
- Visual impairment
- Chronic cardiorespiratory disease
- Injuries and complications of falling
- Problems with feet and footwear.

Careful and accurate assessment is essential with the aim of identifying treatable causes so as to focus the efforts of the multidisciplinary team. Remember that being immobile can lead to further disabling and potentially fatal complications such as pressure sores, hypostatic pneumonia, DVT, osteoporosis, limb contractures, urinary retention and faecal impaction.

Answers

 CASE 6.4 – A 74-year-old man who has difficulty walking is referred to the elderly medicine day hospital.

 Q1: What is the differential diagnosis?

A1

- Cervical myelopathy
- Gravitational and calcium antagonist-induced lower limb oedema
- Infected leg ulcers
- Possible DVTs.

 Q2: What features in the history support the diagnosis?

A2

The history of neck surgery for arthritis and the finding of UMN signs in the arms and legs (with no evidence of neurological dysfunction above the neck) is highly suggestive of cervical myelopathy consequent upon degenerative disease of the cervical spine.

Impaired mobility, obesity and dependency of the lower legs will predispose to venous stasis, oedema and ulceration (and in due course infection). This is a potent setting for venous thrombosis. Calcium antagonists can exacerbate peripheral oedema caused by venous dilatation.

Urinary incontinence is inevitable in this setting owing to immobility and impaired bladder control caused by compression of the cervical spinal cord.

 Q3: What additional features in the history would you seek to support the potential diagnoses?

A3

- History of neck trauma or injury or arthritic symptoms with acute-on-chronic deterioration requiring neurosurgical intervention.
- Constipation: common in this setting and exacerbated by calcium antagonists.
- History of previous venous thrombosis or peripheral vascular disease (PVD).
- Symptoms of breathlessness or chest pain (pulmonary embolism [PE]).

Q4: What other features would you look for on clinical examination?

A4

- Signs of PE or heart failure

- Pressure sores (buttocks, sacrum, heels)

- Faecal impaction and urinary retention

Q5: What investigations would you perform?

A5

- Full blood count (FBC): infection

- Renal function and plasma glucose: renal failure and diabetes mellitus

- Urinalysis:

  – heavy proteinuria if oedema caused by nephrotic syndrome

  – glycosuria

  – protein and blood consistent with urinary infection

- Midstream specimen of urine (MSU): infection

- Leg ulcer swab and blood cultures: to guide antibiotic therapy

- Venous and arterial Doppler studies of legs: detection of venous thrombosis and exclusion of ischaemic leg ulceration

- Cervical spine radiograph: cervical spondylosis/osteoarthritis

- Magnetic resonance imaging (MRI) of cervical spine: to detect spinal cord compression

- Chest radiograph and ECG: heart failure and pulmonary embolism.

Q6: What treatment options are available?

A6

- Neck surgery for cervical myelopathy is unlikely to be successful in this setting as a result of chronicity of symptoms. Surgery could also be very hazardous as a result of significant co-morbidity.

- Elevation of legs to diminish oedema.

- Antibiotics for cellulitis.

- Compression bandaging or hosiery to control peripheral oedema once cellulitis has resolved and arterial ischaemia excluded.

- Pressure relief mattress/cushion to areas at high risk of pressure sores.

- Anticoagulant therapy if venous thrombosis confirmed (consider DVT prophylaxis if absent).

- Discontinuation of calcium antagonist. Consider an alternative agent such as a diuretic (but might exacerbate incontinence), an ACE inhibitor (might impair renal function) or a β blocker (care if heart failure/diabetes present).

- Treatment for heart failure if confirmed.

- Attention to bowel and bladder function.

- Referral to multidisciplinary team for rehabilitation and resettlement at home in due course.

CASE 6.5 – You have been called to see a 72-year-old man who lives alone at home.

 Q7: What investigations would you perform?

A7

Basic investigations should include:

- Hip radiograph essential: osteoarthritis or avascular necrosis of femoral head or fractured neck of femur

- FBC: secondary polycythaemia, infection

- Renal function tests: uraemia and electrolyte imbalance

- Measurement of ABGs should be considered because of the signs of respiratory failure and possible hypercapnia

- Chest radiograph and ECG: to support the diagnosis of chronic obstructive pulmonary disease (COPD) and cor pulmonale

- Peak expiratory flow rate (PEFR) and/or spirometry before and after inhaled bronchodilator will confirm COPD and determine the degree of reversibility.

Q8: What treatment options are available?

A8

Management is going to be difficult at home as a result of the need for radiographs and specialist tests, and the presence of respiratory failure. Hospital admission is advisable in order to confirm the diagnoses and assess the degree of respiratory failure. Time will be needed for rehabilitation and adaptations to the home environment.

Treatment will be along the following lines:

- Analgesia for osteoarthritis (avoiding opiates and non-steroidal anti-inflammatory drugs [NSAIDs] if possible – potential respiratory depression and fluid retention respectively)

- Bronchodilators, controlled oxygen and cautious use of diuretics for COPD and cor pulmonale

- Laxatives and enemas for faecal impaction/constipation

- In due course, consideration of hip replacement if the patient is agreeable and cardiorespiratory status permits.

Q9: What are the likely causes of his immobility?

A9

- Osteoarthritic hip: a hip fracture is less likely as a result of the chronicity of the symptoms and absence of trauma.

- COPD (chronic bronchitis and emphysema) and cor pulmonale.

- Urinary incontinence caused by immobility is almost inevitable in this situation, perhaps exacerbated by coexisting prostatism or faecal impaction.

 Q10: What can be done to improve his situation at home?

A10

Much depends on the potential to improve and the feasibility of hip surgery. Even so, adaptations to the home with appropriate seating and bedding, as well as a review of toilet and washing arrangements, will be necessary. His ability to climb stairs safely will need to be assessed. He will need assistance with shopping and other household tasks. A multidisciplinary team approach is required to resolve these various issues, including physiotherapy, occupational therapy and social worker involvement. An early discharge might be achieved with forward planning and utilization of domiciliary rehabilitation services.

● **CASE 6.6 – A 68-year-old, previously active, woman is now unable to walk or stand having sustained a stroke (right middle cerebral artery territory infarction) 3 weeks previously.**

Q11: What treatment options are available?

A11

Depression is common at this stage and can seriously interfere with rehabilitation. An antidepressant in conjunction with psychological support and a positive approach by the multidisciplinary team can help alleviate this.

- Anticoagulants: there is a risk of further stroke (12–15 per cent per annum), which can be reduced by two-thirds after anticoagulation with warfarin (international normalized ratio [INR] 2.0–3.0).

- Anti-embolic stocking: will help to diminish the risk of DVT and lower limb oedema.

- Laxative: to prevent constipation.

- Analgesia: pain and stiffness are common in this situation.

- ACE inhibitor: if BP persistently > 140/80 mmHg (but be vigilant about the risk of precipitating symptomatic postural hypotension in this setting).

Q12: In addition to regular medical and nursing attention, which members of the multidisciplinary team ought to be involved with her care?

A12

- Physiotherapist: to prevent contractures, maintain posture, avoid shoulder injury and improve function.
- Occupational therapist: to promote independence and overcome functional impairments caused by motor, sensory and visual impairments.
- Speech and language therapist: including assessment and therapy to improve swallowing.
- Dietitian: modification of diet to enhance safe swallowing and maintain adequate hydration and nutrition.
- Stroke nurse specialist/psychologist: specialist advice, support and counselling to both patient and family.
- Social worker: to explore any social issues relevant to a timely, safe and supported discharge from hospital.

Q13: What medical complications might supervene during the next 4–6 weeks?

A13

- Painful shoulder caused by joint subluxation or capsular/rotator cuff injury (correct manual handling essential to minimize this complication)
- DVT/PE
- Pneumonia (aspiration or hypostatic)
- Urinary tract infection (UTI)
- Faecal impaction
- Pressure sores
- Limb contactures
- Depression
- Post-stroke epilepsy
- Recurrent stroke (haemorrhagic transformation or re-infarction).

👥 OSCE Counselling Cases – Answers

OSCE COUNSELLING CASE 6.3 – A 75-year-old man who lives in a nursing home is confined to his bed or chair owing to a previous left-sided stroke.

A1

Areas include the following:

SKIN CARE AND PRESSURE AREAS

- Pressure sores (especially sacrum, hips and heels)
- Intertrigo in skin folds such as groins, axillae and perineum
- Leg ulcers complicating dependent oedema of the lower limbs
- Soft tissue infections.

BLADDER AND BOWELS

Urinary incontinence is inevitable in this situation and will necessitate regular toileting and/or containment by pads, sheath drainage or (as a last resort) urinary catheterization. Urinary catheter care will include regular catheter changes (3 to 4 monthly) to prevent encrustation, blockage and leakage.

Bowel function will need review. Faecal incontinence, constipation and faecal impaction with overflow diarrhoea might all need appropriate management.

NUTRITION

Obesity will exacerbate nursing difficulties. On the other hand, difficulty swallowing, resulting in poor nutrition, might cause weight loss. Provision of food and drink of appropriate consistency and manoeuvres to improve swallowing will need discussion. Nutritional and vitamin supplementation might prove necessary. Liaison with dietitian and speech and language therapist might also be helpful.

LIMB CONTRACTURES/OEDEMA

- Flexion contractures of the limbs can develop over time and can be ameliorated to some extent by appropriate positioning of the hemiplegic limb, as well as physiotherapy and anti-spasticity drugs such as baclofen.
- Dependent oedema and DVT can develop in an immobile lower limb. Elastic hosiery can help to prevent this.
- Shoulder pain can develop as a result of incorrect handling/lifting techniques.

RESPIRATORY COMPLICATIONS

Aspiration and/or hypostatic pneumonia.

MEDICATION REVIEW

The need for laxatives, analgesics, hypnotics and the appropriateness of medication for secondary stroke prevention (aspirin, a statin, antihypertensives) will need periodic review.

SOCIAL AND PSYCHOLOGICAL WELL-BEING

Good quality care should encompass this important area too. Apathy and depression are common after a disabling stroke. Boredom and isolation can lead to difficult behaviour. Regular visits from friends and family should be facilitated. Interest in former hobbies and pursuits should be encouraged as far as is possible. Social activities, access to radio, TV, etc. are also important, being mindful of the patient's preferences and interests. Advice from a speech and language therapist will be helpful in order to maximize communication.

OSCE COUNSELLING CASE 6.4 – A 65-year-old woman is reviewed in clinic after recent colonic surgery.

The essence to this case is to discuss risk reduction and distinguish this from prevention. DVT is a well-recognized problem post-surgery. The risk is higher in those with prothrombotic states (such as malignancy or a hypercoagulable syndrome, e.g. factor V Lieden mutation) and where venous return may be compromised (pelvic surgery, lower limbs raised intraoperatively, e.g. lithotomy position or with a pneumoperitoneum – laparoscopic surgery).

To try to prevent this, patients will be given a low-molecular-weight (LMW) heparin, are preoperatively well hydrated with intravenous fluids (especially if they have had preoperative bowel preparation), will be wearing thromboembolic deterrent stockings and may have been asked to stop any prothrombotic medication before surgery (e.g. tamoxifen). (LMW heparin works by activating anti-thrombin III; it inhibits platelet aggregation and decreases the availability of thrombin. It has a longer half-life than heparin and therefore requires only a single daily administration. The fact that its response is much easier to predict removes the need for monitoring.) During surgery the legs are slightly elevated to aid venous return and intermittent calf compression can be used. Post-surgery, early mobilization is encouraged.

Even with these precautions there is still a risk of a DVT developing. The importance of making the diagnosis and treating appropriately should be emphasized.

If there has been an aberration to the normal protocols, increasing her risk, it should be admitted and a reason sought. There is often a reason that can be explained (e.g. not giving heparin preoperatively if an epidural is to be inserted). Did the preoperative consent discuss the risk of DVT?

OSCE COUNSELLING CASE 6.5 – The wife of an elderly man is distressed because her husband's attendance at the local elderly care day hospital for physiotherapy has been discontinued.

This is a difficult situation and the decision has probably been made because the patient is not making progress with rehabilitation. A feeling of abandonment heightens the wife's sense of distress at the withdrawal of therapy by the multidisciplinary team. This situation can be avoided or ameliorated in a number of ways:

● Setting clear goals for rehabilitation with realistic time scales that are understood by family/carers and when possible the patient too.

- A graded reduction in therapy, transferring the emphasis of care into more socially oriented activities such as former hobbies and interests

- Ongoing support from a stroke nurse or another member of the multidisciplinary team such as social worker or home-care assistant

- Recognition of the needs of the carer. Attendance at the day hospital might have been a lifeline for the wife in terms of providing regular respite from caring. Alternative arrangements such as a carer to sit with the patient at home or his attendance at a local day centre or stroke club might be helpful.

ACUTE CONFUSIONAL STATES

Q1: List the most likely causes of his or her confusional state
Q2: What initial investigations should you perform?
Q3: What treatment would you consider appropriate?
Q4: The niece is worried about her aunt returning home alone at the conclusion of the hospital admission.
How would you address this concern? (Case 6.9 only)

Clinical cases

● CASE 6.7 – **You have been asked to see an 83-year-old man who has been brought to A&E.**

He lives in a residential home, and for the last 2 days he has become confused. He is not eating or drinking and his walking has deteriorated. He has Parkinson's disease, a history of angina and type 2 diabetes mellitus. His medication includes co-beneldopa, selegiline, gliclazide, a nitrate preparation and aspirin.

On examination the significant findings are as follows:

- Abbreviated mental test: 4/10; he is agitated and restless

- His tongue is dry

- BP 108/62 mmHg

- HR 104/min regular

- His chest is clear

- Marked signs of parkinsonism (rigidity, tremor and bradykinesia)

- Urinalysis: protein ++, blood +, glucose ++ and ketones negative.

● CASE 6.8 – **A 74-year-old man with a history of alcohol abuse was admitted to hospital 24 hours ago after two witnessed epileptic seizures.**

He recovered fully and was initially lucid, but is now very restless and agitated. He seems to be hallucinating. Examination is difficult. He has a low-grade fever, and is tremulous and sweating. There are no obvious focal neurological signs. He is not jaundiced or anaemic. BP 178/84 mmHg; HR 106/min, AF.

● CASE 6.9 – **An 84-year-old woman is found wandering in the street at night by the neighbours and is brought to hospital.**

She is very disorientated and confused. She is alert, but restless and agitated. She is convinced that she is late for work. A telephone call to her niece confirms that the patient has been somewhat confused and forgetful for the last 9 months or so. Further enquiry reveals that she needs help with her household and financial affairs. She has never wandered before.

Examination discloses AF (126/min), cardiomegaly, mitral incompetence and peripheral oedema. Her feet are in a state of neglect and there is an infected bunion. Abbreviated mental test is 4/10. There are no focal neurological signs. The remainder of the examination is unremarkable. Q3 is not applicable in this case.

🏃 OSCE Counselling Cases

OSCE COUNSELLING CASE 6.6 – What advice should be given to the matron of a local nursing home who telephones the local GP reporting that one of her elderly residents, who has Alzheimer's disease, has become uncharacteristically agitated and restless?

OSCE COUNSELLING CASE 6.7 – An 84-year-old woman has been brought to A&E having been found wandering at night.

She is alert but confused (Mini-Mental State Examination [MMSE] 12/30 (normal 27+/30). There are no focal neurological signs, but she is cold (core temperature 35.5°C). She is unable to give a coherent history. You telephone her daughter to gain more historical information.

List five key aspects of the history that you need to establish in discussion with the daughter.

🔑 Key concepts

In order to work through the core clinical cases in this section, you will need to understand the following key concepts.

Acute confusion or delirium is a syndrome not a diagnosis and can be the mode of presentation of almost any illness, especially in elderly people. The most important question is 'why?' There is great danger (for lack of collateral history) in assuming that the patient has 'always been like this' or even that only one factor is involved. Always search for multiple pathology.

Common precipitating factors include:

- Infections

- Metabolic disturbances (e.g. hypo- or hyperglycaemia, dehydration, electrolyte imbalance, uraemia, hypothermia)

- Hypoxia and/or heart failure

- Pain or injury

- Surgery and anaesthesia

- Drugs (especially anticholinergic, dopaminergic or opiate therapy and alcohol/tranquillizer withdrawal states)

- Sensory overload (e.g. unfamiliar surroundings or situations)

- Pre-existing cognitive impairment (often mild and previously unnoticed) or sensory impairment (deafness and/or poor vision) is a common predisposing factor in older people, producing an 'acute-on-chronic' confusional state.

The cornerstone of management is to detect and correct the underlying causes as well as general measures to re-orientate and reassure the patient. Sedation should be considered only when agitation/confusion is preventing essential tests or treatment, the patient's behaviour poses a danger to him- or herself or others, or it is necessary to relieve severe distress in an agitated patient. The maxim 'start low and go slow' when prescribing for older patients is particularly germane in this setting.

Answers

 CASE 6.7 – **You have been asked to see an 83-year-old man who has been brought to A&E.**

 Q1: List the most likely causes of his confusional state

A1

His confusional state is multifactorial. Precipitating factors might include: UTI, dehydration and hyperglycaemia. Drugs, selegiline (a monoamine oxidase type B inhibitor [MAOI-B]) and levodopa, (medications prescribed for treatment of Parkinson's disease) can also precipitate confusion, particularly in susceptible patients, i.e. those with pre-existing cognitive impairment. Other potential factors might include silent MI (hypotension and history of coronary artery disease) or stroke (symptoms and signs difficult to elicit owing to confusion and agitation). Enquiry about falls and head injury (even trivial) is important because of the potential for subdural haematoma.

 Q2: What initial investigations should you perform?

A2

- FBC: infection

- Sepsis screen: urine and blood cultures as well as chest radiograph

- Renal function tests: electrolyte imbalance and uraemia

- Plasma glucose: to assess diabetic control

- C-reactive protein (CRP) or erythrocyte sedimentation rate (ESR): non-specific markers of an inflammatory or infective process

- ECG: MI

- Arterial oxygen saturation: to identify hypoxaemia caused by cardiopulmonary disease.

 Q3: What treatment would you consider appropriate?

A3

- Rehydration (intravenous) and correction of electrolyte disturbance

- Sliding scale insulin infusion for control of diabetes

- Broad-spectrum antibiotic to cover UTI (after obtaining appropriate cultures)

- Discontinue selegiline: this drug is more likely to precipitate confusion than L-dopa-based medications

- Maintain co-beneldopa at the minimum dose required to control parkinsonian symptoms

- General measures to reassure and re-orientate the patient

● Prevention of falls and pressure sores

● Avoid major tranquillizers (haloperidol, etc.), which, in the presence of Parkinson's disease, might precipitate a severe neuroleptic sensitivity reaction.

● CASE 6.8 – A 74-year-old man with a history of alcohol abuse was admitted to hospital 24 hours ago after two witnessed epileptic seizures.

Q1: List the most likely causes of his confusional state

A1.

Alcohol withdrawal causing delirium tremens is very likely given the time course of his confusional state. Hypoglycaemia might also be present, given the history of alcohol abuse and the potential for liver disease.

Occult head injury should also be considered. Inebriated or fitting patients are at great risk of injury and will have little, if any, recollection of the event. Older patients with alcohol abuse are particularly susceptible to subdural intracranial bleeding as a result of the combined effects of trauma, cerebral atrophy and coagulopathy.

The history of seizures raises the possibility of an intracranial space-occupying lesion (e.g. subdural haematoma, tumour), although either alcohol excess or withdrawal itself can precipitate seizures. Electrolyte imbalance, particularly hyponatraemia (syndrome of inappropriate antidiuretic hormone secretion [SIADH]), must be considered in the setting of head injury or intracranial space-occupying lesion.

● Infection: pneumonia, meningitis, urine are all possibilities in this setting.

● Liver encephalopathy is unlikely in the absence of jaundice.

● A check for gastrointestinal bleeding (per rectum) is important (note sweating and tachycardia), although the elevated BP mitigates against this.

Q2: What initial investigations should you perform?

A2

● Capillary glucose: hypoglycaemia

● Plasma U&Es: SIADH

● Liver function tests (LFTs) and INR: liver damage and synthetic liver function

● FBC: bleeding and infection

● Blood cultures; urine dipstick and culture should be sent as soon as a sample can be obtained

● Chest radiograph when feasible: pneumonia

● Arterial oxygen saturation: hypoxia

● CT of head: space-occupying lesion/bleeding

Lumbar puncture should be considered (meningitis?) if the above tests fail to identify a cause and there is no evidence of space-occupying lesion, bleeding or raised intracranial pressure on CT of the brain and no coagulopathy.

Q3: What treatment would you consider appropriate?

A3

Delirium tremens is very likely and should be treated with a benzodiazepine (e.g. intravenous diazepam followed by oral chlordiazepoxide) tapered over 3–4 days.

Intravenous thiamine is also advisable because malnourished individuals with alcohol problems are at risk of developing Wernicke's encephalopathy.

Intravenous glucose (50 mL 25 per cent dextrose i.v.) if hypoglycaemia is detected on capillary glucose reading (send plasma sample to lab for confirmation, but do not delay treatment while awaiting result).

Once agitation and confusion have been controlled, careful clinical examination is needed to assess for other causes of confusion as outlined above.

CASE 6.9 – An 84-year-old woman is found wandering in the street at night by the neighbours and is brought to hospital.

Q1: List the most likely causes of her confusional state

A1

The history is very suggestive of an acute-on-chronic confusional state, the former precipitated by acute illness(es). Underlying cognitive impairment as a result of early Alzheimer's diseases is quite likely in this setting but must not be assumed. A search for acute illnesses such as infection (urine, infected bunion, respiratory), side effects of medication, heart failure and metabolic disturbance (diabetes, uraemia, etc.) is essential. She is wandering at night so hypothermia must be considered.

In addition to an acute illness, causes of chronic confusion must be considered such as dementia (Alzheimer's or vascular brain disease), thyroid dysfunction, vitamin B_{12} deficiency and hypercalcaemia. If there is a poorly maintained gas appliance at home, chronic CO poisoning might need to be excluded.

Q2: What initial investigations should you perform?

A2

- FBC: anaemia, infection

- Urinalysis and MSU: infection, diabetes

- Blood cultures and swab e.g. from infected bunion

- Plasma electrolytes, glucose and renal function: metabolic disturbance and uraemia

- Calcium: confusion caused by hypercalcaemia

- Thyroid function tests: often difficult to interpret in acute illness, but in this case important to exclude thyroid dysfunction, particularly hyperthyroidism in view of AF and heart failure

- Chest radiograph: infection, heart failure

- ECG: to confirm AF

- Arterial oxygen saturation (and spectrophotometry for carboxyhaemoglobin if CO poisoning suspected)

Once the acute illnesses have settled and if chronic confusion persists, CT of the brain should be considered to exclude potentially treatable causes of chronic confusion such as hydrocephalus, meningioma and chronic subdural haematoma. Vitamin B_{12} and folate levels are needed if there is macrocytic anaemia.

Q4: The niece is worried about her aunt returning home alone at the conclusion of the hospital admission. How would you address this concern?

A4

This is a difficult issue and there is insufficient information provided to formulate an answer to this question. Once acute confusion has settled cognitive and functional status should be reassessed by the multidisciplinary team (occupational therapist and social worker, in particular). An old age psychiatry consultation might be required, particularly if dementia is confirmed, so that an assessment of mental capacity can be made. If the patient insists on returning home alone, a judgement about her capacity to assess the risk involved will be important. Assessment of the patient's home environment will also be important before a decision about discharge is finalized. Acetylcholinesterase inhibitor therapy, given to enhance cognition, is contraindicated in this case because of cardiac disease.

♟♟ OSCE Counselling Cases – Answers

OSCE COUNSELLING CASE 6.6 – What advice should be given to the matron of a local nursing home who telephones the local GP reporting that one of her elderly residents, who has Alzheimer's disease, has become uncharacteristically agitated and restless?

This is a common scenario often referred to as an acute-on-chronic confusional state. Older people with impaired cognitive reserve are at greater risk of delirium and this is often precipitated by events such as intercurrent illness (commonly infection), an adverse reaction to medication, emotional distress or pain/discomfort. The first priority is to ensure the patient's safety while identifying and correcting the offending precipitant.

The nurses should check for symptoms and signs of common infections such as UTI (fever, dysuria, incontinence, abnormalities on urinalysis) and respiratory infection (cough, wheezing, dyspnoea). The medication chart should be reviewed to see whether there are any new medications or amended dosages. Physical distress resulting from urinary retention, faecal impaction, pain from injury (any recent fall?) or emotional upset should be identified and corrected. If there is any suspicion of underlying medical illness, a prompt medical assessment will be needed.

In the interim, the nurses should be advised to monitor the patient unobtrusively and enhance orientation by ensuring adequate soft lighting, to ensure that any hearing aid is operational and that spectacles are worn. A calm, confident approach is needed and the reassurance of a close family member or friend is helpful.

The nurses should be asked to watch the patient closely to prevent accidents and injury, while encouraging fluids to correct or prevent dehydration.

It is likely that the confusional state will settle if the offending precipitant is identified and corrected, although it might take a few days or sometimes longer for the older person to settle back to normal. In many instances a hospital admission (with its attendant hazards to a frail older person) can be avoided, but this will require close cooperation of the doctor, nursing staff and family/carers.

OSCE COUNSELLING CASE 6.7 – An 84-year-old woman has been brought to A&E having been found wandering at night.

1. Duration of confusion

2. Systems enquiry

3. Previous medical history

4. Drug history

5. Social history.

DURATION OF CONFUSION

Is this an acute, acute-on-chronic or chronic confusional state? The first two conditions, i.e. acute or acute-on-chronic confusion, warrant a diligent search for intercurrent general medical conditions that might have precipitated the current delirious state (e.g. infection, CNS event such as head injury, metabolic disturbance, hypothyroidism). The latter condition, i.e. chronic confusion (duration > 6 months), is more consistent with a dementing illness such as Alzheimer's disease.

SYSTEMS ENQUIRY

The patient cannot give a coherent account of events, but while lucid might have previously reported important symptoms to a close relative or carer. Enquiry along these lines might reveal, for example, a description of a recent head injury (subdural haematoma), urinary symptoms (infection), thirst and urinary frequency (diabetes mellitus), or cold intolerance (hypothyroidism), etc.

PREVIOUS MEDICAL HISTORY

This might give important information relevant to the current presentation, e.g. a history of liver disease, cerebrovascular disease, chronic renal impairment or cardiopulmonary disease might cause or predispose to an acute confusional state.

DRUG HISTORY

Medications can commonly cause of confusion in older patients. Offending agents include: anticholinergics (e.g. trihexyphenidyl for Parkinson's disease), tricyclic antidepressants (e.g. amitriptyline), opiates, hypoglycaemic agents (e.g. glibenclamide) and dopaminergic drugs (e.g. L-dopa). Alcohol should also be considered.

SOCIAL HISTORY

This information is essential in order to gain a proper understanding of the context of the presenting illness, potential for rehabilitation and, in due course, discharge planning.

INCONTINENCE

? Questions for the clinical case scenarios given

Cases 6.10 and 6.11
Q1: What are the likely causes of the problem?
Q2: How should the problem be investigated?
Q3: What can be done to help?
Case 6.12
Q4: What are the likely causes of the problem?
Q5: What treatments should be considered?
Q6: Suggest three reasons why the incontinence has gone unreported by the patient for so long

Clinical cases

● CASE 6.10 – A 78-year-old woman, disabled by stroke, is cared for by her daughter.

Care at home is proving difficult as a result of persistent urinary incontinence such that a nursing home placement is now being considered. The patient has a left hemiparesis and dysphasia, and needs help to stand, transfer and walk. She receives treatment with aspirin (for stroke), amlodipine (for hypertension) and furosemide (for swollen ankles).

The patient is alert and responsive, but has difficulty communicating as a result of her dysphasia. Sometimes she is able to indicate that the lavatory is needed, but is usually wet before toileting can be achieved.

In addition to the signs of stroke, examination shows an excoriated perineum. There is no palpable bladder. Rectal examination is normal. There is no uterovaginal prolapse.

● CASE 6.11 – An 82-year-old man with advanced Parkinson's disease and dementia is cared for in a nursing home.

His nursing needs are usually fairly predictable. Of late, he has become more agitated than usual. He seems uncomfortable and has started to shout and rattle the bedsides, and occasionally he hits out at the nurses. The on-call GP has prescribed a sedative to settle the patient at night. He is continuously wet with urine and, unusually for him, is now incontinent of liquid faeces too. He has no fever and other vital signs are normal.

● CASE 6.12 – A 90-year-old woman who lives alone has slipped and fallen in her bathroom at home.

She has escaped serious injury. Subsequent visits by the district nurse to assess the situation reveal that the elderly woman's clothing is always soaked in urine and the house has a strong smell of urine. The patient is reluctant to discuss the situation but does admit to a swelling 'down below'. She is sensible and independent in her activities of daily living. She is reluctant to be examined by the nurse, but in due course assessment reveals a swelling at the vaginal introitus, which on further examination is shown to be the cervix. When the patient stands up she leaks urine. Her bowel function is normal.

There are no other abnormal findings. In particular there is no palpable bladder, neurological examination is normal and urinalysis is negative.

👥 OSCE Counselling Cases

OSCE COUNSELLING CASE 6.8 – An elderly hypertensive woman is attending the surgery for regular assessment of her BP.

On this occasion her daughter attends as well and mentions that the family is very concerned about the patient's apparent incontinence of urine. The daughter goes on to say that her mother's house and clothing have now developed a constant smell of urine. On direct questioning the patient makes light of this problem. She seems sensible.

How would you proceed?

OSCE COUNSELLING CASE 6.9 – An 86-year-old woman is distressed by persistent incontinence of urine.

Outline the key steps to establishing the cause of this problem in a primary care setting.

🔑 Key concepts

In order to work through the core clinical cases in this chapter, you will need to understand the following key concepts.

Urinary incontinence to some degree is common in elderly people, affecting about 12 per cent of men and 20 per cent of women aged 65 and over, compared with 1 per cent and 6 per cent of those aged 15–64 years. Transient causes include confusional states, immobility, urine infection, diabetes, stroke, retention with overflow and drugs. Incontinence can persist if the above conditions remain unresolved. Established incontinence can also occur in many other chronic disorders. Examples include: unstable bladder resulting from detrusor instability (urge incontinence), pelvic floor incompetence (stress incontinence), neurogenic bladder (e.g. spinal cord lesions, cerebrovascular disease), as well as incontinence associated with dementia, prostatism, bladder tumour or stone, and of course immobility from any cause.

Assessment must include a full history and examination, including per rectum and (if appropriate) per vaginam, as well as CNS and locomotor assessments. Investigations include urinalysis, MSU, U&Es, glucose, calcium, plain abdominal radiograph and/or ultrasonography and, in selected patients, urodynamic studies.

Accurate diagnosis and treatment are essential. Effective treatments for urge incontinence include bladder retraining and drugs to stabilize the bladder (e.g. anticholinergics such as oxybutynin and tolterodine), but side effects can be problematic in elderly people. Stress incontinence can be helped by pelvic exercises to strengthen the pelvic floor as well as surgical suspension procedures. Devices to ameliorate incontinence (pads, sheath drainage, urinals, intermittent self-catheterization) are effective to varying degrees and are appropriate steps to avoid permanent catheterization with its attendant hazards (infection, soreness, bypassing, etc.).

Faecal incontinence is less frequent than urinary incontinence, but can be more distressing to the patient and carers. Community-based studies reveal a 2 per cent prevalence of faecal incontinence in people aged over 65 years, rising to about 25 per cent in the over-85-year age group. Prevalence rates in nursing homes and hospital is even higher. In a British study, only half those reporting faecal incontinence had discussed this with a health-care professional. Causes include underlying diseases in the rectum or anus (e.g. tumour), faecal impaction with overflow diarrhoea (secondary to immobility caused by, for example, stroke or arthritis), neurological disorders affecting sphincter control (similar to those causing urinary incontinence) and cognitive disorders such as dementia or severe depression. Once again accurate diagnosis and treatment of remedial factors are essential (e.g. enemas for faecal impaction). When remedial measures fail or are inappropriate, faecal incontinence can be controlled by means of a drug-induced constipation regimen alternating with periodic planned bowel evacuation by enema or suppository.

Answers

 CASE 6.10 – A 78-year-old woman, disabled by stroke, is cared for by her daughter.

 Q1: What are the likely causes of the problem?

A1

In this situation there are several factors responsible for the urinary incontinence:

- Damage to the CNS by a stroke will have impaired the central capacity to inhibit bladder (detrusor) contractions, resulting in frequency and urgency of micturition.

- Immobility as well as difficulty calling for help and perhaps cognitive dysfunction will precipitate urinary incontinence.

- Diuretic therapy will exacerbate the need to pass urine quickly.

- Immobility and incomplete bladder emptying both predispose to UTIs which can also cause incontinence.

Q2: How should the problem be investigated?

A2

- Urinalysis and MSU: to assess for infection, diabetes or occult renal disease

- U&Es: hypokalaemia, hyponatraemia and renal failure

- Plasma glucose: polyuria caused by hyperglycaemia

- FBC: infection.

 Q3: What can be done to help?

A3

- Discontinue the diuretic and observe. There is no history or signs of heart failure. Ankle swelling is a common side effect of calcium antagonist medication such as amlodipine. If this can be withdrawn, diuretic therapy might no longer be required. Persisting hypertension might be better managed by a β blocker or ACE inhibitor. In this situation, elastic hosiery is a more appropriate method for controlling dependent oedema.

- Assess communication and cognition with the help of a speech and language therapist. Try to improve the patient's ability to communicate the need to pass urine (bell, picture card, gestures, etc.).

- There should be an assessment of the home environment and toilet facilities by an occupational therapist. Techniques to allow clothing to be removed quickly, assistance with transfers as well as equipment to facilitate toileting (commode, grab rails, raised toilet seat, etc.) will promote continence.

- District nurse and carer to work with the patient to establish a regular toileting regimen so as to anticipate and thus prevent incontinence. Pads and barrier cream are needed to protect the perineum.

- Antibiotics if UTI confirmed.

- If the above measures prove insufficient, consider stabilization of the bladder with anticholinergic medication, e.g. tolterodine or oxybutynin. Such treatment needs to be used with caution because of predictable anticholinergic side effects (confusion, glaucoma, constipation, dry mouth, etc.).

- Finally, assistance with toileting and washing at home from the home-care service and regular monitoring of the situation by the district nursing team. Regular respite care should be considered to sustain the daughter in her caring role.

CASE 6.11 – An 82-year-old man with advanced Parkinson's disease and dementia is cared for in a nursing home.

Q1: What are the likely causes of the problem?

A1

Urinary and faecal incontinence are not uncommon in the setting of dementia and relative immobility caused by conditions such as Parkinson's disease. Nevertheless, regular toileting and maintenance of a daily bowel habit by appropriate diet, simple laxatives and, when necessary, suppositories, are usually sufficient to maintain control of this situation. In this scenario, it is very likely that faecal impaction has supervened with overflow of liquid stool. This is a most uncomfortable situation for the elderly man who is unable, as a result of confusion, to draw attention to his predicament. Urinary retention with overflow of urine is also very common in this setting, particularly if there is pre-existing urinary outflow obstruction as a result of prostatic enlargement. Anticholinergic drugs, sometimes used (inappropriately) in older patients with Parkinson's disease, and opiate-based analgesics can also precipitate this problem.

Urinary infection is not infrequent in this setting, but would usually be associated with fever and offensive urine. Infective diarrhoea would tend to produce profuse liquid stool associated with fever and dehydration and there might also be other affected residents in the home. *Clostridium difficile* enteritis should be considered if the patient has recently received a broad-spectrum antibiotic.

Q2: How should the problem be investigated?

A2

- A careful clinical examination (even if difficult) is essential, with particular reference to fever, hydration, bladder enlargement (often non-tender in chronic retention) and rectal examination (prostatic enlargement and/or impaction with hard stool).

- Urinalysis and, if appropriate, stool culture for evidence of infection.

- Plasma U&Es should be sent if obstructive uropathy or dehydration is suspected.

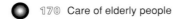 Q3: What can be done to help?

A3

Faecal impaction should be relieved by regular enemas, with attention to regular bowel care as outlined in A1. Once constipation is relieved, urinary retention might resolve spontaneously – especially if the patient is able to sit or stand to pass urine. Failing this, temporary urinary catheterization (with measurement of residual urine to confirm the diagnosis) should be performed until the bowel function has normalized. Anticholinergic- and/or opiate-based medication should be withdrawn. Treatment for UTIs should be guided by antibiotic therapy. Infectious diarrhoea will require 'barrier nursing' precautions to prevent the spread of infection. *C. difficile* enteritis should respond to oral metronidazole or vancomycin.

● CASE 6.12 – **A 90-year-old woman who lives alone has slipped and fallen in her bathroom at home.**

 Q4: What are the likely causes of the problem?

A4

The patient has a third-degree uterine prolapse resulting in stress incontinence as a result of pelvic floor (sphincter) incompetence. A history of leakage of urine when straining, coughing, laughing or even standing is usual. There is a recognized relationship between stress incontinence and weakness of pelvic floor musculature and sphincter tone. Ageing, oestrogen deficiency, previous multiparity and surgical interference at parturition are also predisposing factors.

 Q5: What treatments should be considered?

A5

Lesser degrees of pelvic floor incompetence can be treated to good effect by pelvic floor exercises taught by a physiotherapist, in conjunction with oestrogen replacement therapy. The situation described in this scenario requires gynaecological referral and control of uterine descent by either pessary or surgery.

 Q6: Suggest three reasons why the incontinence has gone unreported by the patient for so long

A6

Incontinence is often unreported by older patients. Embarrassment, social isolation, and fear of investigation or treatment and acceptance as 'normal' ageing or that 'nothing can be done' are all factors to a greater or lesser degree.

👥 OSCE Counselling Cases – Answers

OSCE COUNSELLING CASE 6.8 – An elderly hypertensive woman is attending the surgery for regular assessment of her BP.

Urinary incontinence is a common problem in old age and is often unreported. The reasons for this reluctance to seek medical advice are multi-factorial and include embarrassment, a belief that nothing can be done or that it is an inevitable consequence of ageing. Health-care professionals can also fail to enquire about this symptom or, if it is mentioned, may feel unable to intervene in an effective manner.

The first step is to secure the patient's confidence and trust. An approach by the practice nurse might be a more successful first step in order to gain an initial history and preliminary assessment. It will be important for the nurse/doctor to emphasize that assessment is relatively simple and that an effective treatment is very likely. Even if cure is not feasible, improvement and/or containment of symptoms is certainly possible.

The initial assessment should include a thorough history and examination (note rectal and vaginal examinations), paying particular attention to medications as well as any gynaecological and/or neurological symptoms and signs. Urinalysis, urine culture and bladder scan (to assess bladder emptying and residual volume) are also essential steps in the assessment. Most assessments can be completed in a general practice setting and measures instituted to improve the common conditions of urge and stress incontinence. The advice of a continence nurse specialist is useful for the treatment of complex cases and where a more detailed knowledge of containment devices and pads is required.

OSCE COUNSELLING CASE 6.9 – An 86-year-old woman is distressed by persistent incontinence of urine.

KEY STEPS

The key steps include a full history focusing on:

- Precipitating factors

- Pattern of voiding, including assessment of frequency and volume

- Previous as well as current medical and surgical illnesses, including obstetric procedures and problems

- Drug history especially diuretics, anticholinergics, sedatives, opiates

- Assessment of functional status and toileting arrangements

- Corroborative details from carer/relative.

FULL EXAMINATION

Full examination focusing on:

- Abdomen: for retention of urine, pelvic masses

- Rectal examination: for constipation, tumour, anal tone

- Vaginal examination: for prolapse, tumour, atrophic changes

- Full neurological assessment: searching for evidence of cognitive dysfunction and other CNS diseases, such as stroke, Parkinson's disease, spinal cord disease, autonomic dysfunction.
- Locomotor examination.

INVESTIGATIONS

Simple, focused investigations in response to the findings on history and examination, including:

- Urinalysis
- MSU
- Measurement of residual volume (by catheterization or ultrasonography)
- Capillary glucose
- Plasma urea creatinine and electrolytes
- Plain radiograph of kidneys, ureters and bladder (for renal/bladder stone).

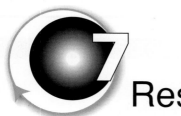

Respiratory medicine

Malcolm Shepherd and Neil C. Thomson

DYSPNOEA

? **Questions for each of the clinical case scenarios given**

Q1: What is the likely differential diagnosis?
Q2: What issues in the given history support the diagnosis?
Q3: What additional features of the history would you seek to support a particular diagnosis?
Q4: What clinical examination would you perform and why?
Q5: What investigations would be most helpful and why?
Q6: What treatment options are appropriate?

Clinical cases

● CASE 7.1 – Episodic breathlessness and wheeze.

A 35-year-old mother attends the medical outpatient clinic complaining of breathlessness with wheeze. This can occur at rest and has been getting worse over the last 2 years. Between episodes of breathlessness she feels better but does not feel that she ever returns to 'normal'. Occasionally she awakens with shortness of breath and coughing in the early hours of the morning.

● CASE 7.2 – Chronic dyspnoea and cough.

A 66-year-old retired publican attends the respiratory outpatient clinic complaining of severe exercise limitation as a result of breathlessness. He has trouble moving about the house and rarely goes outside. He feels worse in the mornings and describes wheeze. His symptoms have developed over 3 years and his GP has tried inhalers but they have not helped. He has had a cough with sputum for more than 10 years. He has been a smoker for more than 40 years and has smoked 5–10 cigarettes per day over this time.

● CASE 7.3 – Progressive dyspnoea and weight loss.

A 66-year-old man presents complaining of worsening exercise tolerance as a result of breathlessness. He can walk 200 metres on a flat road whereas 1 year ago he could manage at least 1 mile. He also describes feeling short of breath at rest. He is severely restricted on hills or stairways. He denies cough, but has lost 3 kg over the last 6 months. He is a life-long non-smoker and worked in the ship-building industry where he was exposed to asbestos fibres. His GP describes inspiratory crackles at both lung bases.

♟♟ OSCE Counselling Case

OSCE COUNSELLING CASE 7.1 – **A 72-year-old man who suffers from cryptogenic fibrosing alveolitis attends the clinic with his daughter. They both feel that he requires oxygen to help him with his daily activities.**

A 72-year-old man who suffers from cryptogenic fibrosing alveolitis (CFA) attends the clinic with his daughter. They both feel that he requires oxygen to help him with his daily activities.

Q1: What criteria should you assess before prescribing oxygen?

Q2: What advice would you give to him about the use of oxygen?

☛ Key concepts

In order to work through the core clinical cases in this chapter, you will need to understand the following key concepts.

Spirometry

This is a useful test that is quick to perform and has good reproducibility. Spirometry measures the volume and velocity of a forced exhalation over approximately 5 seconds. Two important values are derived. First, the volume of air expired in the first second, known as the forced expiratory volume in 1 s (FEV_1), and, second, the total volume exhaled in the 5 s, the forced vital capacity (FVC). In the context of dyspnoea two patterns are frequently found. If both values are lower than predicted for an individual's size, age and gender, the pattern is described as a 'restrictive pattern' whereas if the FEV_1 is disproportionately smaller than the FVC, i.e. FEV_1/FVC ratio ≤ 75 per cent, the pattern is known as an 'obstructive pattern'.

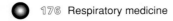

Answers

 CASE 7.1 – Episodic breathlessness and wheeze.

 Q1: What is the likely differential diagnosis?

A1

- Asthma
- Hyperventilation
- Recurrent pulmonary embolism (PE).

 Q2: What issues in the given history support the diagnosis?

A2

Episodic breathlessness, wheeze and cough with spontaneous resolution are typical of asthma. Symptoms tend to occur at night, first thing in the morning or after exercise but none of these clinical features is specific for asthma. Progression over 2 years may suggest insufficient treatment of asthma.

Q3: What additional features of the history would you seek to support a particular diagnosis?

A3

A smoking history should be taken. It would be useful to assess likelihood of other associated atopic diseases by enquiring about allergic rhinitis and eczema. Any environmental or other factors that exacerbate her breathlessness should be identified, e.g. occupational asthma. A chronic cough without wheeze either currently or in the past may suggest cough variant asthma.

 Q4: What clinical examination would you perform and why?

A4

Examination is likely to be normal unless the patient is suffering from an exacerbation.

General examination should look for evidence of eczema, (dermatitis, ichthyoid skin). Respiratory examination may reveal wheeze or hyperinflated lung fields.

Q5: What investigations would be most helpful and why?

A5

- Peak expiratory flow (PEF): this is the most useful objective test to try to confirm a diagnosis of asthma. A 2-week recording of the PEF measured twice a day can identify diurnal variation that is characteristic of asthma ($\geq$ 20 per cent from baseline). Specific but insensitive diagnostic test.

- Spirometry: a single measurement may be normal or may demonstrate a low FEV_1/FVC ratio (an obstructive pattern). An improvement in FEV_1 of > 15 per cent and 200 mL after inhalation of a bronchodilator or a 2-week course of corticosteroid therapy is highly suggestive of asthma.

- Chest radiograph: unhelpful in diagnosing asthma but may rule out alternative diagnoses or pneumothorax.

- Full blood count (FBC): not useful although blood eosinophilia may occur occasionally in asthma

- RAST (radioallergosorbent test), IgE to common allergens: these tests may identify specific agents to which the patient is sensitive that could trigger asthmatic reactions. Common allergens include cat or dog hair, house-dust mite and grass pollen.

 ## Q6: What treatment options are appropriate?

A6

- Assess asthma control: pattern and severity of symptoms and exacerbations, supplemented where appropriate with serial PEF recording. An oral steroid trial (as above) may be required to demonstrate the patient's best spirometry.

- Eliminate trigger factors.

- Patient education: ensure understanding of medications and how to alter treatment in the event of deterioration, and check inhaler technique. Provide a written asthma action plan.

Stepwise drug treatment:

- Step 1: mild intermittent asthma – inhaled short-acting β_2 agonist as required.

- Step 2: regular preventer therapy – add inhaled steroid 200–800 μg daily for patients with recent exacerbations, nocturnal asthma or using short-acting β_2 agonists more than once daily.

- Step 3: add-on therapy – add inhaled long-acting β_2 agonists agonist twice daily.

- Step 4: persistent poor control – increase inhaled steroid dose up to 2000 μg daily, or consider trial of leukotriene receptor antagonist, theophylline preparation or oral β agonist.

- Step 5: continuous or frequent use of oral steroids – use daily steroid tablets in lowest dose tolerated.

CASE 7.2 – **Chronic dyspnoea and cough.**

Q1: What is the likely differential diagnosis?

A1

● Chronic obstructive pulmonary disease (COPD)

● Asthma

● Bronchiectasis.

 Q2: What issues in the given history support the diagnosis?

A2

Chronic progressive breathlessness on the background of a long smoking history suggests COPD. Typical features include lack of spontaneous improvement or response to inhaled therapy, relentless progression of symptoms and a combination of productive cough and dyspnoea. Although he has only a 20 pack-year smoking history, his occupation and the variable effects of cigarette smoking make COPD the most likely diagnosis.

Q3: What additional features of the history would you seek to support a particular diagnosis?

A3

A history of previous reversible wheeze and dyspnoea might suggest chronic asthma. Productive sputum can accompany bronchiectasis and predisposing features should be sought, e.g. childhood infections. Assessment of severity in terms of lifestyle and exercise impairment should be made. Chronic lung disease can precipitate depression and the patient's mood should be assessed because antidepressants can help.

Q4: What clinical examination would you perform and why?

A4

Physical examination is rarely diagnostic in COPD. Look for signs of respiratory failure (central cyanosis), hypercapnia (bounding high-volume pulse, flapping tremor) and/or cor pulmonale (raised jugular venous pressure [JVP], ankle or sacral oedema). Physical signs of airflow obstruction usually occur only when severe airflow obstruction is present, e.g. pursed lipped breathing, hyperinflated thorax, paradoxical in-drawing of intercostal spaces, resonant percussion note, poor breath sounds or wheeze.

Q5: What investigations would be most helpful and why?

A5

- Spirometry: baseline spirometry with reversibility to bronchodilators should be performed in all patients suspected of having COPD. The FEV_1 is typically < 80 per cent of the predicted value, and the FEV_1/FVC ratio is < 70 per cent; these values do not return to normal with a bronchodilator. A short course of oral steroids can be used to help distinguish chronic asthma from COPD. Post-bronchodilator FEV_1 is used to classify the severity of COPD.

- Chest radiograph: no specific features, but upper zone emphysema, hyperinflation (more than six ribs anteriorly), and flattened diaphragm would support the diagnosis. It is useful to exclude an alternative diagnosis such as bronchial carcinoma.

- Arterial blood gases (ABGs)/pulse oximetry: measure in patients with severe disease; oxygen saturation ≤ 92 per cent should lead to ABG measurement.

- FBC: useful to exclude anaemia or polycythaemia.

- α_1-Anti-trypsin: may identify deficiency in rare cases; check in patients aged under 45 years.

 Q6: What treatment options are appropriate?

A6

- Aims of management: to lessen dyspnoea, reduce exacerbations and improve exercise tolerance with minimal side effects.

- Reduce risk factors: smoking cessation is the most effective way to reduce the risk of developing COPD and stop its progression.

- Bronchodilators: although no objective improvement in spirometry is seen in response to bronchodilator therapy in COPD, patients may derive symptomatic benefit. They should therefore be provided with inhaled bronchodilators, either a short-acting β_2 agonist or anticholinergic therapy. Patients with more severe symptoms should be given a trial with an inhaled long-acting β_2 agonist or anticholinergic agent. Other agents may be tried on a symptomatic trial basis, including oral theophyllines.

- Inhaled steroids: result in small reductions in the frequency of exacerbation in severe COPD. Combination therapy of an inhaled long-acting β_2 agonist and an inhaled steroid may reduce the frequency of exacerbations more effectively than either drug alone.

- Oxygen therapy: long-term oxygen therapy is recommended for patients who have stopped smoking and who have chronic respiratory failure (PaO_2 < 7.3 kPa).

- Pulmonary rehabilitation: useful to maximize patient functional capacity.

- Immunization: against influenza yearly.

- Depression: mood assessment should be made with intervention where appropriate.

CASE 7.3 – Progressive dyspnoea and weight loss.

 Q1: What is the likely differential diagnosis?

A1

- CFA
- Pulmonary asbestosis
- Cardiogenic pulmonary oedema.

 Q2: What issues in the given history support the diagnosis?

A2

Progressive dyspnoea in a non-smoker with no history of cough may suggest fibrotic (interstitial) lung disease. Dyspnoea is frequently first encountered on effort, but progression to dyspnoea at rest is common. The history of occupational exposure to asbestos may suggest an industrial component to this disease, but formal diagnosis requires further investigations. Crackles are typical of some forms of interstitial lung disease and are frequently confused with pulmonary oedema.

Q3: What additional features of the history would you seek to support a particular diagnosis?

A3

An attempt should be made to quantify the degree of functional impairment experienced by the patient. The degree of exposure to asbestos fibres should be enquired about. The history should also include information on any systemic disease, drug therapy, travel and environmental exposures, e.g. agents known to cause extrinsic allergic alveolitis (EAA) such as bird protein or mouldy hay. A history of ischaemic heart disease (IHD) or hypertension makes pulmonary oedema more likely.

 Q4: What clinical examination would you perform and why?

A4

General examination should look for evidence of respiratory or cardiac failure. Ankle oedema, cyanosis, tachycardia and respiratory rate should all be examined. Finger clubbing is frequently associated with CFA but less often in asbestosis. Respiratory examination may reveal poor thoracic excursion, normal percussion note and widespread inspiratory crackles. Weight loss frequently accompanies interstitial lung disease, but assessment for bronchial carcinoma should be made.

Q5: What investigations would be most helpful and why?

A5

- Chest radiograph: may be normal or reveal shrunken lungs with coarse vascular markings (honeycomb lung) or patchy areas of consolidation. Evidence of asbestos exposure may be found such as pleural calcification or plaques.

- High-resolution computed tomography (HRCT): may reveal long-standing changes of fibrosis (honeycombing) or the more acute changes associated with active inflammation (ground-glass intra-alveolar shadowing).

- Pulmonary function tests: typically a 'restrictive' pattern of spirometry would be expected (FEV_1/FVC ratio normal, but both values less than predicted). Total lung volumes and static volumes are reduced and CO diffusion gradient is also reduced.

- Oxygen saturation/tension: it is useful to assess the degree of hypoxaemia, because this helps to quantify the severity of disease and may indicate patients who will benefit from the administration of domiciliary oxygen therapy. A 6-minute walk test with S_{O_2} (oxygen saturation) measurements is a sensitive test of early interstitial lung disease.

- Serum markers of EAA: serum precipitins to avian proteins and other causes of EAA should be sought.

- FBC: of little use although an elevated haematocrit may develop in response to chronic hypoxia.

- Autoimmune antibodies: these may reveal the coexistence of connective tissue diseases that may present with interstitial lung disease such as rheumatoid arthritis, systemic lupus erythematosus (SLE) or systemic sclerosis.

 Q6: What treatment options are appropriate?

A6

- General: patients should avoid any causal agents. Advice on seeking industrial compensation is appropriate in the case of pulmonary asbestosis.

- Drug treatment: controlling the progression of pulmonary fibrosis may be achieved in CFA by systemic corticosteroid therapy or immunosuppressive treatment, although the response to treatment is often disappointing. Domiciliary oxygen may be prescribed for patients with end-stage disease.

♔♔ OSCE Counselling Case – Answer

OSCE COUNSELLING CASE 7.1 – **A 72-year-old man who suffers from CAF attends the clinic with his daughter. They both feel that he requires oxygen to help him with his daily activities.**

A1

SOCIAL CRITERIA

There is concern over the use of oxygen supplementation in the context of possible exposure to naked flame. Oxygen can promote combustion and may make house fires more likely. It is recommended that patients who smoke are not prescribed oxygen and that oxygen is not used in homes heated by open flame fires.

PATIENT CRITERIA

● Assess requirement: patients with interstitial pulmonary disease may benefit from oxygen as a palliative measure at later stages of the disease. The degree of alveolar hypoxia should be estimated by ABG measurement and the secondary consequences of hypoxaemia should be assessed. If PaO_2 is < 8 kPa and symptoms of dyspnoea are disabling to the patient, oxygen may be prescribed on an 'as required' basis.

● Assess capacity: oxygen is administered from either constant flow cylinders or from concentrators each of which must be delivered to the patient's home. The patient's capacity to use the device should be assessed and where necessary training or additional support from, for example, specialist nursing service should be arranged.

A2

There is concern over the safety of over-reliance on domiciliary oxygen. Patients should be advised that oxygen is safe in stable respiratory disease, but that it is not a substitute for medical intervention in the event of a sudden deterioration. Therefore if dyspnoea gets worse despite normal use of oxygen, medical advice should be sought.

There is concern about excess oxygen in COPD. Patients who have COPD may become dependent on hypoxic drive to stimulate respiration, and COPD can complicate many respiratory conditions including fibrosing alveolitis. Although supplementary oxygen is safe if properly assessed, increasing the supply of oxygen may depress respiratory drive. Patients are advised not to make changes to the flow settings on their concentrators or cylinders, without seeking advice.

PLEURITIC CHEST PAIN

? Questions for each of the clinical case scenarios given

Q1: What is the likely differential diagnosis?
Q2: What issues in the given history support the diagnosis?
Q3: What additional features of the history would you seek to support a particular diagnosis?
Q4: What clinical examination would you perform and why?
Q5: What investigations would be most helpful and why?
Q6: What treatment options are appropriate?

Clinical cases

● CASE 7.4 – Sudden pleuritic chest pain and haemoptysis.

A 35-year-old woman is brought to the accident and emergency department (A&E) complaining of acute onset of chest pain the preceding evening and collapsing that afternoon. She is shocked and dyspnoeic. This pain is described as 'sharp', located posteriorly on the left hemithorax, and worse on inspiration and coughing. On the morning of admission there was some haemoptysis. She has recently been in hospital for treatment and investigation of recurrent miscarriage.

● CASE 7.5 – Gradual-onset pleuritic chest pain and haemoptysis.

A 73-year-old man attends his GP complaining of left-sided, 'sharp' chest pain. The pain is worse on inspiration, does not radiate and has appeared in the last 2 days. He has not felt well for 1 week with uncontrollable shivering bouts and sweats. He has had a cough with red-tinged sputum for 3 days. He smokes 20 cigarettes a day, and has angina complicated by a myocardial infarction (MI) 2 years previously. He has recently felt increasingly short of breath with effort.

● CASE 7.6 – Sudden pleuritic chest pain and dyspnoea.

A 30-year-old man attends A&E complaining of chest pain and breathlessness. The pain developed suddenly, 16 hours before attendance, and he has gradually become increasingly short of breath since. The pain is described as sharp, worse on inspiration or coughing, and located on the right thoracic chest wall. He denies new cough or sputum production.

⚄ OSCE Counselling Case

OSCE COUNSELLING CASE 7.2 – A 35-year-old woman has completed 6 months of anticoagulation therapy after having a life-threatening pulmonary embolus. She now wonders if she should consider oral contraception rather than risk further pregnancy.

This 35-year-old woman was finally diagnosed as having a life-threatening PE. Having received 6 months of anticoagulation therapy she returns to her doctor for advice. Her main concerns surround whether she should now consider oral contraception rather than risk further pregnancy.

Q1: What risks exist and how should the GP advise her?

⚯ Key concepts

In order to work through the core clinical cases in this chapter, you will need to understand the following key concepts.

Pleuritic pain

This is pain usually localized to the thoracic wall, whose severity varies with respiration. Thus typically the pain will be worse on inspiration and relieved by expiration. Commonly coughing exacerbates this type of pain. It normally derives from inflamed layers of pleura moving over each other.

Thromboembolism

This is the passage of blood clots from a peripheral source to a more proximal vascular bed. Typically the origin of thromboembolism is the deep veins of the leg and clots frequently lodge in the pulmonary arterial circulation.

Community-acquired pneumonia

This title distinguishes infective pneumonia that has developed in the community from those conditions that develop in a hospital setting. These conditions are caused by different organisms and carry different prognoses.

Additional factors associated with pulmonary thromboembolism (PTE)

Pre-test probability (PTP) scores: these are designed to calculate the numerical risk of PE, based on clinical assessment, to guide the interpretation of more detailed investigation. Such scores include the presence of tachypnoea (respiratory rate or RR > 30), tachycardia, chest pain, clinical evidence of deep venous thrombosis (DVT), abnormal ECG (as a new finding) and abnormal chest radiograph. The presence of one or more clinical feature plus one of the baseline investigations is said to have a sensitivity for PE of > 80 per cent.

Additional features in community-acquired pneumonia

British Thoracic Society (BTS) guidelines: assessment of confusion (each question scores 1 mark, maximum score 10 marks):

- Age
- Date of birth
- Time (nearest hour)
- Year
- Hospital name
- Recall address (e.g. 24 West Street)
- Date of First World War
- Name of monarch
- Count backwards from 20
- Recognition of two people (e.g. doctor or nurse)

A score of 8 or less = mental confusion

Answers

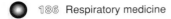 CASE 7.4 – Sudden pleuritic chest pain and haemoptysis.

 Q1: What is the likely differential diagnosis?

A1

- PE
- Community-acquired pneumonia with septic shock
- Tension pneumothorax.

 Q2: What issues in the given history support the diagnosis?

A2

Pleuritic chest pain with dyspnoea and haemoptysis is typical of PE. A recent spell in hospital where she may have been relatively immobile and the history of recurrent miscarriages, which may be associated with thrombophilia, are potential risk factors for PE. The sequence of a small embolic event followed by a more clinically significant episode with haemodynamic compromise is typical of PE.

 Q3: What additional features of the history would you seek to support a particular diagnosis?

A3

Further enquiry should attempt to identify risk factors for DVT, e.g. smoking, history of DVT, PE or malignancy, recent long-haul airline flight, family history of DVT or PE, and recent surgical procedures and use of DVT prophylaxis. A history of leg swelling may indicate current DVT.

Q4: What clinical examination would you perform and why?

A4

The clinical presentation demands urgent emergency assessment and should follow the standard advanced life support (ALS), ABC (A for airway, B for breathing and C for circulation) protocol.

Further clinical assessment should be aimed at identifying the presence of DVT and assessing the severity of respiratory and haemodynamic compromise. Thus the respiratory rate, pulse rate, blood pressure (BP) and presence of cyanosis should be recorded. Calves should be examined for swelling or tenderness and any circumferential differences should be measured and documented. Detailed respiratory examination including auscultation, which may reveal localized wheeze, a pleural rub or be normal, should be performed. A loud pulmonary second heart sound is rarely heard in acute PE.

Q5: What investigations would be most helpful and why?

A5

- Chest radiograph: may be normal, show oligaemia or pleural-based wedge-shaped shadowing.

- ECG: tachycardia, atrial fibrillation, rarely S1, Q3, T3 pattern.

- Oxygenation: either saturation or PaO_2 by arterial puncture is useful to assess severity.

- Blood D-dimers: have high negative predictive value; measure only when there is a reasonable suspicion of PE.

- CT pulmonary angiogram (CTPA): has replaced pulmonary angiogram as the imaging of choice.

- Ventilation/perfusion isotope lung scan: normal scans reliably exclude PTE. Positive or negative scans are diagnostic in between 30 and 50 per cent of cases, but rely on a normal chest radiograph appearance

- Thrombophilia screen: important in this case given the history of recurrent miscarriage. Protein S, protein C, von Willebrand's factor, lupus anticoagulant and factor V Leiden should all be measured.

 Q6: What treatment options are appropriate?

A6

- Assessment: the initial management of this patient depends on the degree of haemodynamic compromise.

- Immediate steps should be made to stabilize her condition, including supplementary oxygen therapy, intravenous fluid resuscitation and transfer to a location where intensive monitoring can be performed.

- If she remains haemodynamically unstable, thrombolytic therapy should be administered intravenously. Thrombolysis is the first-line treatment for massive PE.

- If the patient is stable: a pre-test probability of PE should be made before investigation and further management should be directed by the likelihood of PE based on this PTP score and the appropriate investigations. If clinical suspicion of PTE is high, full-dose anticoagulation should be initiated with low-molecular-weight (LMW) heparin, while oral anticoagulant therapy (warfarin) is commenced at a loading regimen. Anticoagulation should be continued for a minimum of 6 months and discontinued if there are no obvious predisposing factors remaining. Consideration to life-long therapy should be made in the light of ongoing risk factors.

● CASE 7.5 – Gradual-onset pleuritic chest pain and haemoptysis.

 Q1: What is the likely differential diagnosis?

A1

- Community-acquired streptococcal pneumonia

- Community-acquired pneumonia caused by 'atypical pathogen'

- PE

- Tuberculosis (TB).

Q2: What issues in the given history support the diagnosis?

A2

Symptoms typical of infection (fevers or sweats) with pleuritic chest pain suggest pneumonia; however, they can be associated with PE. Although there are no clinical features specific for a given pathogen, *Streptococcus pneumoniae* remains the most common cause of community-acquired pneumonia. The so-called 'atypical' pathogens such as *Mycoplasma* species, *Legionella pneumophila* and *Chlamydia* species represent a substantial minority. In this patient, the age, the presence of pleuritic chest pain and the cardiovascular co-morbidity are all associated with streptococcal infections. The red-tinged or rusty sputum is said to typify streptococcal infections, but haemoptysis may occur with other pulmonary infections, especially TB.

 Q3: What additional features of the history would you seek to support a particular diagnosis?

A3

Co-morbid conditions, associated with a poor outcome in community-acquired pneumonia should be sought, e.g. diabetes mellitus, cystic fibrosis or chronic lung disease. If the patient has been bedridden or confused since the onset of symptoms his prognosis is worse. It is very difficult reliably to determine the cause of pulmonary infections by history alone. Contact with TB should be enquired after.

Q4: What clinical examination would you perform and why?

A4

Clinical examination in community-acquired pneumonia is directed at confirming the diagnosis and measuring a severity score. The latter informs management decisions, including the best location for treatment (home, ward or intensive care unit [ICU]), and the likely prognosis.

General examination should identify cachexia, pyrexia (the absence of fever in community-acquired pneumonia carries a poor prognosis), cyanosis and peripheral lymphadenopathy, and the presence of labial herpes simplex. A Mini Mental State Examination (MME) should be performed and recorded (a score of < 8/10 is associated with a poor prognosis). Respiratory rate, pulse rate and BP should be recorded. Respiratory examination should look for the typical features of consolidation, including dull percussion note, bronchial breathing, increased vocal fremitus and whispering pectoriloquy.

 Q5: What investigations would be most helpful and why?

A5

Investigations are used to confirm the diagnosis and assess likely prognosis.

- Chest radiograph: the most useful investigation in confirming the diagnosis. Unfortunately no single feature can identify the causative organism. Multi-lobar involvement and/or pleural effusions are more frequent in bacteriological pathogens and cavitation is more common with *Staphlococcus aureus* or *Klebsiella pneumoniae* infections. Multi-lobar involvement carries a poor prognosis.

- FBC: high leukocytosis (> 20 × 10⁹/L) or leukopenia (< 4 × 10⁹/L 9) carries a poor prognosis.

- Urea and electrolytes (U&Es): a high urea has a worse prognosis and renal failure suggests severe sepsis.

- Liver function tests (LFTs), creatine kinase: commonly abnormal in legionella infections.

- Sputum culture: unless previous antibiotics have been administered.

- Blood cultures and sensitivities: a very sensitive marker for aetiology if positive.

- Serum for serology: paired samples for atypical serology

- Urine and blood samples: for pathogen antigens.

 Q6: What treatment options are appropriate?

A6

Assessment: initial management decisions should be informed by a severity assessment score. No such scores have been fully validated, but the CURB-65 is commonly used. This score addresses **c**onfusion (described as an MMSE of < 8/10), serum **u**rea elevated > 7, **R**R > 30/min, abnormal **B**P (systolic < 90 mmHg, diastolic < 60 mmHg) and age > **65** years. Community treatment is likely to be safe if none or one of these markers is present; the presence of two or more requires hospital assessment and may require admission either to a ward or an ICU setting.

Treatment: medical treatment should include:

- supplementary oxygen if required

- the administration of intravenous fluids

- the administration of antibiotic therapy.

Initially an empirical choice is required; however, this should not be delayed because the time to first dose of antibiotic correlates with outcome. It is rare to have sufficient clues as to the identity of the infecting organism to guide initial choice. In the UK most streptococcal infections remain sensitive to β-lactam antibiotics, whereas most atypical organisms are sensitive to macrolides. It is reasonable therefore to prescribe co-amoxiclav and clarithromycin in the first instance, and await sensitivities or treatment failure to guide further selection. In a hospital setting an initial intravenous dose and a choice of intravenous or oral medication thereafter is frequently used. In the community both penicillin and macrolide antibiotics are well absorbed orally.

 CASE 7.6 – Sudden pleuritic chest pain and dyspnoea.

 Q1: What is the likely differential diagnosis?

A1

- Left-sided pneumothorax

- PE.

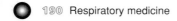

 Q2: What issues in the given history support the diagnosis?

A2

Sudden onset of chest pain suggests either trauma or spontaneous pneumothorax. As no history of a precipitating event is given spontaneous pneumothorax is the most likely diagnosis. Frequently the pneumothorax will enlarge over time and thus dyspnoea may develop relatively late. Pulmonary embolus should always be considered; however, there is no supporting history given.

 Q3: What additional features of the history would you seek to support a particular diagnosis?

A3

The previous history of similar events is important because recurrent disease (even if not picked up clinically) is likely to lead to further episodes and will usually be treated by a definitive procedure. Employment history is important because professional diving or flying is banned after a pneumothorax. Recreational diving is also not recommended and should be enquired about.

Q4: What clinical examination would you perform and why?

A4

- Assessment of severity: ABC (A for airway, B for breathing and C for circulation). Occasionally pneumothoraces may develop 'tension' and precipitate haemodynamic compromise. Cyanosis, tachycardia, hypotension and evidence of mediastinal shift (away from the side of the chest pain) are indications of severity. Respiratory examination may reveal tracheal shift (away from pneumothorax), hyperresonant percussion note on the side of the pneumothorax and normal on the opposite side; reduced or normal breath sounds may be present.

- Assessment for predisposing conditions: this should be made, e.g. Marfan's syndrome may present with pneumothorax and so it is worth examining arm span, palate and eyes for lens dislocation, and carefully for an ejection systolic murmur.

Q5: What investigations would be most helpful and why?

A5

- Chest radiograph: although, if clinical suspicion of tension pneumothorax is high, treatment should not await radiological examination

- Oxygenation: either saturation (if > 93 per cent) or ABGs

- FBC: not useful in a pneumothorax

- U&Es: not useful in a pneumothorax

- Cardiac echocardiogram: if clinical suspicion of aortic incompetence (in Marfan's syndrome).

Q6: **What treatment options are appropriate?**

A6

- If haemodynamic compromise: immediate puncture of the chest wall in the second intercostal space anteriorly with a large bore Venflon, releasing air from the pleural space. Attach a 50 mL syringe and a three-way tap after release of air and perform underwater sealed aspiration of remaining air.

- If no compromise and chest radiograph confirms the diagnosis: the first step is to perform aspiration under water seal. If there is no obvious predisposing lung disease this should be sufficient to treat the pneumothorax. This procedure is less likely to be successful if there is underlying disease such as COPD or bullous disease (secondary pneumothorax).

- Failed aspiration or secondary pneumothorax: chest drain insertion and attached to underwater seal to allow the gradual reinflation of the lung and removal of pleural gas. Administration of supplemental oxygen is said to hasten reabsorption of pleural gas.

- If a second or recurrent pneumothorax is present: a pleural sealing procedure should be performed such as talc pleurodesis or video-assisted pleurectomy.

⚇⚇ OSCE Counselling Case – Answer

OSCE COUNSELLING CASE 7.2 – **A 35-year-old woman has completed 6 months of anticoagulation therapy after having a life-threatening pulmonary embolus. She now wonders if she should consider oral contraception rather than risk further pregnancy.**

Pulmonary embolus is a rare condition affecting between 1 and 4/1000 people in the UK per year. This risk is increased in pregnant women tenfold over non-pregnant women. This risk is further increased if known risk factors coexist. Such risk factors include age > 35 years, a thrombophilia, obesity (body mass index [BMI] > 30 kg/m^2), paraplegia or inflammatory bowel disease.

RISKS

In this case the history of life-threatening PE and recurrent miscarriage makes the presence of a thrombophilia more likely. The precise risk depends on the nature of each thrombophilia. This patient carries three risk factors: age, history and a likely thrombophilia.

Advice on further pregnancy: pre-pregnancy advice from a specialist should be sought. Extensive investigation of a thrombophilia is important. Treatment with LMW heparin can be instituted throughout pregnancy, so investigation before pregnancy is helpful.

Advice on contraception: the oestrogen content of the oral contraceptive pill is associated with a thrombotic risk. The history of life-threatening PE contraindicates the oral contraceptive in this case and alternative methods should be used.

HAEMOPTYSIS

Q1: What is the likely differential diagnosis?
Q2: What issues in the given history support the diagnosis?
Q3: What additional features of the history would you seek to support a particular diagnosis?
Q4: What clinical examination would you perform and why?
Q5: What investigations would be most helpful and why?
Q6: What treatment options are appropriate?

Clinical cases

● CASE 7.7 – Two weeks of trivial haemoptysis and weight loss.

A 60-year-old man attends the medical outpatient clinic complaining of 4 weeks of cough productive of white sputum and 2 weeks of haemoptysis. The haemoptysis is described as 'streaks of old blood through the spit', and is trivial in volume. It has remained constant throughout the 2-week period. There is no dyspnoea or chest pain, but he is a life-long smoker. He has noticed his clothes being looser over the previous 6 months and describes a loss of appetite, but denies dysphagia or altered bowel habit. He is easily tired and notices his voice becoming hoarse in the evenings. He is a bookmaker and is married with two daughters, one of whom attends with him. She adds that her father appears slightly confused at times, particularly in the evenings.

● CASE 7.8 – Chronic cough and massive haemoptysis.

A 45-year-old mother of two presents at A&E on a Sunday night complaining of coughing large volumes of fresh red blood for the last 2 days. She estimates that she has coughed up five mugs of fresh blood. She describes a cough with purulent sputum for the last month, but cannot remember a time when she did not have a cough. She frequently receives antibiotics from her GP when the sputum turns green or increases in volume. She has been increasingly breathless for the last 2 weeks, although she has noticed increasing breathlessness for 3 years

● CASE 7.9 – Two months of fevers and haemoptysis.

A 62-year-old man attends the respiratory clinic complaining of worsening cough, spit and haemoptysis. This has been of 2 months' duration and is associated with weight loss, anorexia, fevers, night sweats and purulent sputum. He denies chest discomfort or dyspnoea. He lives alone, smokes 20 cigarettes per day and admits to drinking in excess of 40 units of alcohol per week. As a child he was treated for TB at the same time as his father. He was a welder in a shipyard before being made redundant.

👥 OSCE Counselling Case

OSCE COUNSELLING CASE 7.3 – **A 65-year-old man, recently diagnosed as having mycobacterium TB by sputum examination, is brought to the chest clinic by his daughter.**

She tells you that her father is an alcoholic and returns a large number of anti-TB tablets that have not been taken.

Q1: What are the risks of poor compliance with treatment in 'open TB'?

Q2: What options are available to improve compliance?

Answers

 CASE 7.7 – Two weeks of trivial haemoptysis and weight loss.

 Q1: What is the likely differential diagnosis?

A1

- Bronchial carcinoma

- TB

- Upper respiratory tract infection.

 Q2: What issues in the given history support the diagnosis?

A2

Haemoptysis associated with weight loss suggests a systemic disease of uncertain duration. Bronchial carcinoma may present late with haemoptysis after a lengthy period of weight loss and cough. Smoking is associated with most cases of bronchial carcinoma and a non-smoking history should suggest other causes. Associated features of fatigue are non-specific but frequently associated with pulmonary malignancy, whereas hoarseness and confusion should raise suspicions about complications of the disease such as recurrent laryngeal nerve palsy or SIADH.

Q3: What additional features of the history would you seek to support a particular diagnosis?

A3

Employment with a history of asbestos exposure may support pulmonary malignancy. The cumulative lifetime amount of tobacco smoked should be noted, and the presence of constitutional features of fever and sweating may point towards an infective origin of haemoptysis. Pain is an important complication of bronchial carcinoma and can be effectively palliated. Thus, bone or chest wall pain (suggesting advanced disease) should specifically be addressed. An assessment of quality of life and the World Health Organization's 'performance status' is helpful to decide appropriate future management.

Q4: What clinical examination would you perform and why?

A4

Assessment of peripheral (hand – T1 root) muscle wasting, peripheral lymphadenopathy, hepatic enlargement and any unusual or new skin lesions help to identify distant metastases. Finger clubbing is common, but non-specific. Respiratory examination to identify lobar or lung collapse from a central obstructing tumour (tracheal deviation, apex beat, loss of breath sounds) or pleural metastases (signs of effusion) is helpful for baseline assessment of the extent of disease. An assessment of paraneoplastic syndromes can be helpful, e.g. blood pressure (autonomic neuropathy), skin rash (pigmentation [ACTH] or dermatomyositis) or joint stiffness or discomfort (HPOA – hypertrophic pulmonary osteoarthropathy).

Q5: **What investigations would be most helpful and why?**

A5

- Chest radiograph: most important and may reveal diagnosis and complications.
- Bronchoscopy with lavage or biopsy: important test to provide histology, particularly in central tumours.
- Sputum cytology: largely unhelpful with only a 5 per cent sensitivity.
- Computed tomography (CT): may identify non-carcinoma causes of haemoptysis, help staging and biopsy of peripheral lesions seen on chest radiograph.
- U&Es: helpful to exclude SIADH and assess fitness for treatment.
- Serum calcium: elevated in some cases of bronchial carcinoma.
- Liver function tests (LFTs): to help exclude liver metastases.
- Pulmonary function tests: to assess fitness for thoracic surgery.

 Q6: **What treatment options are appropriate?**

A6

Palliate symptoms: haemoptysis, pain and anxiety.

Treat underlying disease:

- Small cell carcinoma: chemotherapy-based treatment. Either as palliation of symptoms (reduced dose) or with curative intent (full dose). Cisplatin-based regimens are now the usual treatment option.
- Non-small cell carcinoma: chemotherapy regimens are used only to downstage extensive disease and allow more definitive therapy to be instituted. Such options include: surgical resection either pneumonectomy or lobectomy, and radiotherapy, either radical or high-dose palliative.
- Fully palliative radiotherapy for symptomatic control.

 CASE 7.8 – Chronic cough and massive haemoptysis.

Q1: **What is the likely differential diagnosis?**

A1

- Bronchiectasis
- PE
- Pulmonary TB.

Q2: What issues in the given history support the diagnosis?

A2

Chronic productive cough is a feature of bronchiectasis, which occasionally presents with massive haemoptysis. Chest discomfort with haemoptysis may simply be associated with coughing-induced musculoskeletal discomfort, but PE should be considered. A change in the volume or purulence of sputum associated with the constitutional features suggests chest infection, which can herald haemoptysis in bronchiectasis.

 Q3: What additional features of the history would you seek to support a particular diagnosis?

A3

A history of a predisposing condition (childhood pneumonias, whooping cough or measles) should be sought but its absence does not exclude bronchiectasis. Evidence of immunodeficiency might be suggested by recurrent infections outwith the chest. A history of fertility problems, e.g. assisted conception, and bowel irregularities throughout life may suggest cystic fibrosis.

Q4: What clinical examination would you perform and why?

A4

- Initial cardiovascular examination to assess degree of blood loss, and thus pulse rate, BP, evidence of peripheral circulation measured to exclude shock.

- Respiratory examination, particularly crackles in any region of the lungs. Palpation of the painful region to confirm the musculoskeletal nature of the pain. Finger clubbing is not present in most cases of bronchiectasis. Wheeze occurs in 75 per cent, crackles in 60 per cent.

Q5: What investigations would be most helpful and why?

A5

- Chest radiograph: most important; in one series 20 per cent of cases of haemoptysis with a normal chest radiograph had bronchiectasis.

- Bronchoscopy: only if haemodynamically significant volumes of blood or to exclude bronchial carcinoma.

- Sputum: helpful for microbiological identification especially *Pseudomonas* species.

- HRCT: diagnostic investigation of choice with a 87–97 per cent sensitivity and 93–100 per cent specificity.

- Bronchial angiography: helpful if radiological treatment of haemoptysis is warranted.

- FBC: for assessment of anaemia.

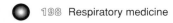 **Q6: What treatment options are appropriate?**

A6

- Resuscitation: if required

- Antitussives: if severe and sometimes also sedation to control cough and anxiety

- Treatment for infection: guided by sputum sensitivities

- Managing haemoptysis: no specific treatment usually; if very severe and persistent consider bronchial artery embolization or, as a last resort, surgical resection.

LONG-TERM MANAGEMENT

Bronchiectasis is a life-long condition that can result in chronic respiratory impairment. Patients should be warned that they might deteriorate over time and require frequent courses of antibiotics. Physiotherapy for lung hygiene may be helpful to reduce the frequency of infective exacerbations and preserve lung function. The evidence for the latter is currently lacking; however, patients should be taught the appropriate exercises tailored to their own specific capacity. Patients should be taught to look out for signs of infection, because prompt and appropriate antibiotic therapy may slow the decline in lung function often associated with bronchiectasis. Specialist therapies may be tried in individual patients, including nebulized antibiotic therapy or long-term rotational antibiotics (in which a series of antibiotics are chronically taken to keep bacterial levels to a minimum with regular changes in the antibiotic to prevent drug resistance).

 CASE 7.9 – Two months of fevers and haemoptysis.

 Q1: What is the likely differential diagnosis?

A1

- TB
- Bronchial carcinoma
- Pneumonia
- Mycetoma
- Bronchiectasis.

 Q2: What issues in the given history support the diagnosis?

A2

A previous history of TB and the consumption of large quantities of alcohol suggest reactivation of old TB. The constitutional symptoms support this diagnosis, but bronchial carcinoma should also be excluded in a smoker with haemoptysis. Previous TB can give rise to mycetoma and bronchiectasis, both of which should be borne in mind. In case series where bronchial carcinoma is rare or excluded, bronchiectasis and TB represent the greatest cause of haemoptysis.

Q3: What additional features of the history would you seek to support a particular diagnosis?

A3

Contact with other people with similar symptoms should be ascertained, as should contact with close family. The type of treatment used for the historical TB may suggest inadequate treatment.

Q4: What clinical examination would you perform and why?

A4

Clinical examination should attempt to exclude TB. Respiratory examination may suggest focal signs of old TB such as crackles in the upper lobes, but may be normal in active TB. Evidence of liver disease should be sought given the alcohol consumption and the possible need for anti-TB therapy.

Q5: What investigations would be most helpful and why?

A5

- Chest radiograph: important
- Sputum: three samples on different days for smears looking for AAFB and culture of organisms (for up to eight weeks)
- Bronchoscopy: to exclude malignancy and allow bronchoalveolar lavage (BAL) and biopsy
- U&Es: baseline
- FBC: assesses anaemia
- LFTs: baseline.

Q6: What treatment options are appropriate?

A6

Assess infectivity and risk:

- Sputum for alcohol- and acid-fast bacilli is an urgent consideration
- Likely contact with children or others. If high risk of contact spread admit for isolation until the sputum is negative for organisms.

DRUG TREATMENT

Assess likelihood of multidrug-resistant (MDR) TB (HIV, foreign contact). If the patient is at high risk, institute quadruple therapy; otherwise triple therapy with rifampicin, isoniazid and pyrazinamide (add ethambutol for quadruple therapy).

It is important in this case also to include pyridoxine and multi-B vitamins to reduce the peripheral neuropathic complications of the anti-TB chemotherapy.

- Assess compliance with therapy – if poor consider directly observed therapy (DOT).
- Contact trace: likely contacts, family members, regular contacts.

♟♟ OSCE Counselling Case – Answers

OSCE COUNSELLING CASE 7.3 – **A 65-year-old man, recently diagnosed as having mycobacterium TB by sputum examination, is brought to the chest clinic by his daughter.**

A1

Tuberculosis diagnosed by sputum examination is likely to be infectious. Although it may be safe to treat this man in the community if his contacts are known, screened and limited, incomplete or no treatment increases the risk to the general public of infectious spread. Before effective antibiotic treatment TB was a fatal disease and failure to take appropriate anti-TB chemotherapy puts the patient's own health at risk. Incomplete or intermittent treatment increases the risk of developing drug-resistant TB. This can lead to chronic infection and the risk of community dissemination of MDR TB.

A2

Alcohol-related liver impairment may worsen the side-effect profile of some anti-TB drugs and may explain his poor compliance. Such a problem should be sought and alternative drugs administered. Usually it is best to admit such a patient to a ward or clinic and reintroduce regular triple therapy in a stepwise manner until the problem can be identified. It is likely that this patient's lifestyle is 'chaotic' and therefore regular compliance with treatment is likely to be poor. In these circumstances DOT may be instituted. Directly observed therapy requires that a trained health-care professional, e.g. TB specialist nurse or equivalent, visits the patient at a prearranged location either daily or on a three times a week basis and observes the treatment being taken. Such practice has been found to reduce the incidence of drug-resistant TB in areas with a relatively high prevalence. In very rare cases compulsory admission can be arranged under public health law. This can be done only in the context of respiratory TB, where there is a considerable risk to the public health. Compulsory administration of medications is not, however, permissible and it is therefore best to develop a concordant rather than a coercive relationship with a patient.

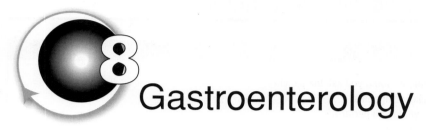

8 Gastroenterology

C.S. Probert

GASTROENTEROLOGICAL EMERGENCIES

? Questions for each of the clinical case scenarios given

Q1: What specific questions would you ask the patient?
Q2: What is the most likely diagnosis?
Q3: What examination would you perform?
Q4: What would be the initial management?
Q5: What investigations would you request to confirm a diagnosis?
Q6: What other issues should be addressed?

Clinical cases

● CASE 8.1 – A 73-year old man with melaena.

A 73-year-old man presents with a 5-day history of passing black stools. On the fifth day he began to feel breathless and tired, particularly on climbing stairs.

● CASE 8.2 – A 26-year old woman with bloody diarrhoea.

A 26-year-old woman presents with a 3-week history of bloody diarrhoea. The blood is fresh and mixed in the liquid stool. Initially, she thought that she might have food poisoning, but could not recall eating anything unusual and had eaten the same food as her unaffected partner.

● CASE 8.3 – A 46-year-old man with alcohol problems and haematemesis.

A 46-year-old man with alcohol problems presents with haematemesis and shock.

ii OSCE Counselling Cases

OSCE COUNSELLING CASE 8.1 – Colitis, is it infectious?

You have determined that the woman in Case 8.2 has ulcerative colitis and tell her that you can treat it. She would like to know whether she could have passed it onto the children in the school where she is a catering assistant.

OSCE COUNSELLING CASE 8.2 – Will my children get it (inflammatory bowel disease)?

The same woman is also worried that she may pass it onto her own children.

Key concepts

In order to work through the core clinical cases in this chapter, you will need to understand the following key concepts.

- Initial assessment of the cause of gastrointestinal (GI) emergencies such as bleeding or severe diarrhoea should be carried out at the same time as resuscitation.

- Most patients with haematemesis and/or melaena will have bled from a peptic ulcer, most cases of which are painless.

- Proton pump inhibitor (PPI) therapy before endoscopic assessment is not evidence based.

- Although stigmata of chronic liver disease may suggest varices as the cause of haematemesis, endoscopic assessment should be made before 'blind' treatment using a Sengstaken–Blakemore tube.

- Any form of colitis may be life threatening.

- Infections should always be sought in parallel with resuscitation with intravenous fluids.

Answers

 CASE 8.1 – A 73-year old man with melaena.

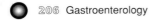 **Q1: What specific questions would you ask the patient?**

A1

The presence of black stools indicates GI bleeding above the ligament of Trietz. The likely sources include benign and malignant ulceration of the stomach and peptic duodenal ulceration. The history should determine whether there are any symptoms suggestive of ulceration, and risk factors and clues to whether the lesion is malignant. Postprandial and nocturnal burning epigastric pains are classic symptoms of peptic ulceration, particularly if the pain radiates to the back. However, these symptoms differentiate poorly between gastric and duodenal ulcers (20 per cent of patients with bleeding peptic ulcers have ulcer-like dyspepsia). Risk factors to seek include:

- Past history of peptic ulceration and/or surgery for such disease

- Recent non-steroidal anti-inflammatory drug (NSAID) ingestion of any type. Warfarin and/or anti-platelet drugs

- Smoking and alcohol

- Diabetes

- Heart failure.

The last three of these are likely to relate to poor mucosal healing. Clues to malignancy include weight loss, anorexia and anaemia before the presenting gastrointestinal haemorrhage.

Q2: What is the most likely diagnosis?

A2

The most likely diagnosis is a bleeding duodenal ulcer. It is unlikely that the patient is bleeding from an oesophageal lesion (carcinoma or oesophagitis) because, in most cases, haematemesis will occur at the same time. Of all patients with acute upper GI bleeding 40 per cent will have benign peptic ulcer disease. Duodenal ulcers appear to be more common than gastric ulcers.

Q3: What examination would you perform?

A3

A full physical examination is necessary with particular attention being paid to shock. However, in a patient of this age, a systolic blood pressure (BP) of 110 mmHg may be considered to be shock. Of secondary importance is the examination of the abdomen during which an epigastric mass and palpable liver should be sought.

Q4: What would be the initial management?

A4

The first step in the management is resuscitation. The patient should be laid flat, given oxygen via a facemask while two large-bore cannulae are inserted, one of which ought to be a central line if the patient is shocked. As the cannulae are inserted, blood samples should be taken for full blood count (FBC), cross-match (4–6 units), urea and electrolytes (U&Es) (as the urea is a marker of the amount of blood lost). Liver function tests (LFTs) are not of immediate importance. Clotting abnormalities need to be sought if the patient is either taking warfarin or has jaundice. Fluid replacement should start as soon as the cannulae are in place. There is no advantage to using colloids. Blood transfusion should start as soon as possible if the patient is shocked or if he has a haemoglobin (Hb) ≤ 10 g/dL. A urinary catheter is desirable.

 Q5: What investigations would you request to confirm a diagnosis?

A5

Oesophagogastroduodenoscopy (endoscopy) should be performed within 24 h of admission. If the patient is shocked or has Hb ≤ 10 g/dL, this should be performed as soon as the patient has been resuscitated, or immediately if urgent surgery is contemplated (i.e. if resuscitation attempts are failing).

 Q6: What other issues should be addressed?

A6

The ulcer is likely to be *Helicobacter pylori* related. Triple therapy should be instituted. This is typically a PPI with two antibiotics from amoxicillin, clarithromycin and metronidazole. If aspirin was being used, then clopidogrel may be substituted.

 CASE 8.2 – A 26-year-old woman with bloody diarrhoea.

 Q1: What specific questions would you ask the patient?

A1

The duration of the disease suggests that the cause is acute colitis. The differential diagnoses include microbial diarrhoea – *Clostridium difficile* (so a drug history is needed) – protozoa (a travel history should be taken), side effects of medications such as NSAIDs, familial adenomatous polyps (the bleeding usually occurs in the context of normal stool – so a family history should be taken). Lifestyle and past medical history should be considered in case the patient is immunocompromised.

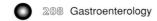

Q2: What is the most likely diagnosis?

A2

The most likely diagnosis is acute colitis, most probably as a result of ulcerative colitis. Other forms of colitis caused by Crohn's colitis, drug side effects or *C. difficile* are possible. Cytomegalovirus (CMV) proctitis and amoebic dysentery are unlikely.

Q3: What examination would you perform?

A3

A full physical examination is necessary with particular attention to examination of the abdomen. Distension and tenderness are particularly worrying physical signs in such a patient. Shock caused by colitis is uncommon, but critically important. Anaemia and a fever should be sought. Severe colitis is defined by the presence of tachycardia, fever and anaemia. Tenderness may indicate toxic dilatation or perforation.

Q4: What would be the initial management?

A4

The patient may require admission or at least discussion with a senior colleague. Assuming that she meets the criteria for admission, i.e. she has severe disease, the initial management includes bedrest, intravenous fluid replacement, hydrocortisone 100 mg i.v. four times daily, transfusion to correct anaemia and nutritional support (typically high-energy food cartons). Heparin is used in most centres: full anticoagulation may treat the disease, whereas prophylactic doses prevent thromboembolism, to which such patients are prone. However, it is important to confirm the diagnosis rapidly. At least three stool cultures should be taken. *C. difficile* toxin must be sought if antibiotics have been consumed recently. Microscopy is often negative, but protozoa must be considered. A plain abdominal radiograph is necessary to assess the diameter of the transverse colon and to look for the distribution of faeces, which may be used to determine disease extent.

Q5: What investigations would you request to confirm a diagnosis?

A5

A limited sigmoidoscopy should be performed by a trained operator. This is a hazardous procedure in untrained hands. However, assessment of the rectal mucosa often helps determine the aetiology of the colitis.

Q6: What other issues should be addressed?

A6

The management of severe ulcerative colitis has two phases: control of the attack and maintenance of remission. If the patient does not respond to intravenous hydrocortisone by the fifth day, a surgical opinion should be sought with a view to colectomy on day 7. Any patient who deteriorates despite intravenous hydrocortisone should also be considered for emergency colectomy. If hydrocortisone controls the attack, the patient should be weaned onto oral steroids and, probably, a 5-acetylsalicylic acid (5-ASA) compound. Steroids should later be discontinued with a view to controlling remission with the 5-ASA compound.

 CASE 8.3 – A 46-year-old man with alcohol problems with haematemesis.

 Q1: What specific questions would you ask the patient?

A1

This is bleeding oesophageal varices until proven otherwise. Although people with alcohol problems may bleed from all the same lesions as those who do not have this problem, any of the former who has bled sufficiently to become shocked is most likely to have varices. If the patient is shocked, treatment must be started before a full history is obtained. Indeed, the patient may be unable to give a history. If a history is available, ask for previous episodes of GI bleeding and treatment for varices.

 Q2: What is the most likely diagnosis?

A2

Bleeding oesophageal varices.

 Q3: What examination would you perform?

A3

Shock should be evaluated quickly: BP, heart rate (HR) and state of peripheral perfusion. Signs of portal hypertension would support the diagnosis: ascites, spider naevi, umbilical hernia. Other evidence of decompensated liver disease should be documented: Glasgow Coma Score (GCS), fetor, flapping tremor and bruising.

 Q4: What would be the initial management?

A4

The patient must be resuscitated as quickly as possible. The patient should be laid flat, given oxygen via a facemask while two large-bore cannulae are inserted, one of which should be a central line. As the cannulae are inserted, blood samples should be taken for FBC, cross-match (4–6 units), U&Es (as the urea is a marker of the amount of blood lost). Albumin and clotting factors (prothrombin time, PT) can be measured to assess synthetic function: other tests, such as alanine transaminase and alkaline phosphatase, assess hepatocyte damage and biliary tract disease/cholestasis, respectively. Synthetic function is an important prognostic indicator. Fluid replacement should start as soon as the cannulae are in place. The central venous pressure (CVP) should be monitored and blood and/or albumin given to maintain a pressure of 10–12 cmH₂O. A urinary catheter is desirable. If the patient is in renal failure, despite an adequate CVP, call for senior help. Vasopressin analogues are desirable, with senior guidance. If the patient remains shocked, a Sengstaken–Blakemore tube may be necessary.

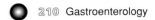

 Q5: What investigations would you request to confirm a diagnosis?

A5

Urgent endoscopy is both diagnostic and therapeutic. This should be performed as soon as the patient is cardiovascularly stable. If such stability cannot be achieved, endoscopy may be performed while resuscitation is continued, provided that the airway is protected.

 Q6: What other issues should be addressed?

A6

Board-spectrum antibiotics should be given because bacteraemia is common at the time of variceal haemorrhage. Anti-encephalopathy treatment (lactulose, metronidazole) should be started as soon as possible. IV thiamine should be replaced before dextrose is given; without this there is a risk of precipitating Wernicke's encephalopathy.

👥 OSCE Counselling Cases – Answers

OSCE COUNSELLING CASE 8.1 – Colitis, is it infectious?

The answer is fortunately 'no'. There are similarities, in the symptoms, between ulcerative colitis and infectious diarrhoea; this is because some infections damage the colon and cause a different kind of colitis. However, infection (in her case) has been ruled out by the stool tests. Furthermore, other tests (sigmoidoscopy ± biopsy) have shown that (her) symptoms are caused by ulcerative colitis.

In the acute phase, most forms of colitis are very similar. Infection should be ruled out in new patients with acute disease.

Three sets of stool analysis are often necessary to exclude *C. difficile* with confidence. Campylobacter infection causes acute colitis with bloody diarrhoea, but myalgia and abdominal pain are conspicuous.

Gastrointestinal infection may occur in patients with ulcerative colitis. Microbiological tests should be performed in patients with an established diagnosis if the attack is atypical or refractory to the usual treatment.

OSCE COUNSELLING CASE 8.2 – Will my children get it (inflammatory bowel disease)?

The answer is fortunately 'no'. Although the disease can appear to run in families the risk is comparatively small. So the chances of the children getting inflammatory bowel disease (IBD) are raised 10 times; the risk is still only 1 in 100, i.e. their chances of getting IBD are less than their risk of diabetes or asthma.

This is an important test of communication skills. The key is to explain relative and absolute risks.

There is a genetic component to the risk of acquiring an IBD. The risk to first- degree relatives is 10–20 times greater than that in unaffected families. However, this raises the prevalence only from 1 in 1000 to 1 in 100.

There is a wealth of literature describing genetic loci in IBD. Although few undergraduates will have read these, all should be aware that loci have been described and that the disease is not sporadic, nor is there a simple mendelian inheritance.

PANCREATITIS

? Questions for each of the clinical case scenarios given

Q1: What specific questions would you ask the patient?
Q2: What is the most likely diagnosis?
Q3: What examination would you perform?
Q4: What would be the initial management?
Q5: What investigations would you request to confirm a diagnosis?
Q6: What other issues should be addressed?

Clinical cases

● CASE 8.4 – A 67-year-old woman with pale stools and weight loss.

A 67-year-old woman presented with diarrhoea. She describes her stools as pale. You discover that she has lost weight, and has nocturia and thirst.

● CASE 8.5 – A 26-year-old woman with abdominal pain and vomiting.

A 26-year-old woman presents with upper abdominal pain and vomiting. Previously she had experienced episodes of right upper quadrant colicky pain that had lasted several hours at a time. On one of these occasions she had experienced a brief episode of jaundice accompanied by dark urine. However, the present episode is different. The pain has lasted for 2 days and appears to be worsening and, this time, it is non-colicky.

● CASE 8.6 – A 48-year-old man with alcohol problems with chronic abdominal pain.

A 48-year-old man with alcohol problems presents with upper abdominal pain with some radiation to the back.

👥 OSCE Counselling Cases

OSCE COUNSELLING CASE 8.3 – 'Why have I got pancreatitis?'

A 26-year-old woman with pancreatitis secondary to gallstones asks 'Why have I got pancreatitis?'

OSCE COUNSELLING CASE 8.4 – 'Why should I stop drinking?'

A 46-year-old man with alcohol problems presents with chronic relapsing pancreatitis asks 'Why should I stop drinking?'

Key concepts

In order to work through the core clinical cases in this chapter, you will need to understand the following key concepts.

- Acute pancreatitis is a significant cause of mortality. It should be considered in the differential diagnosis of all cases of acute abdominal pain.

- The diagnosis can generally be confirmed by an elevated serum amylase.

- Risk factors for acute pancreatitis include alcohol abuse and gallstones.

- Chronic pancreatitis, in general, has an insidious onset.

- Presenting features arise from exocrine failure, later with endocrine failure, accompanied by epigastric pain that usually radiates to the back.

- Diagnosis is reached by assessment of exocrine function and/or imaging.

Answers

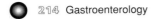

 CASE 8.4 – A 67-year-old woman with pale stools and weight loss.

 Q1: What specific questions would you ask the patient?

A1

The pale stool should prompt questions about malabsorption and/or obstructive jaundice. After asking about jaundice, itching and dark urine – which should all be absent – direct questions to the stool. Look for fluffy, offensive, floating stools. Blood and mucus will be absent. The duration of the symptoms should be noted along with exacerbating and relieving factors. Abdominal pain should be sought – in particular epigastric pain. Such pain is unusual in coeliac disease (although bloating is curiously common), but common in patients with chronic pancreatitis. With regard to the nocturia, assess the volume (small amounts suggest a urinary tract infection [UTI], larger amounts suggest a diuresis – osmotic or drug induced). Large-volume nocturia accompanied by thirst suggests diabetes or hypercalcaemia.

 Q2: What is the most likely diagnosis?

A2

The most likely diagnosis is chronic pancreatitis. This patient exhibits both exocrine and endocrine failure. Pain is absent in 50 per cent of older patients with chronic pancreatitis.

Q3: What examination would you perform?

A3

A full physical examination is necessary with particular attention being paid to the state of nutrition and the cause of the pancreatic failure. Alcoholism and haemochromatosis are associated with signs of liver disease and pigmentation, respectively. However, most patients with alcohol problems have either liver or pancreatic damage. Alcoholism and haemochromatosis are both associated with atrial fibrillation (AF) and cardiomyopathy. A per rectal examination should confirm the colour of the stool.

 Q4: What would be the initial management?

A4

The first step in the management is to corroborate the clinical diagnosis. Blood samples should be taken for calcium, glucose and urea. This will rapidly explain the source of the nocturia. Diabetes should be managed appropriately (see Chapter 1). Early dietetic input should be obtained.

Q5: What investigations would you request to confirm a diagnosis?

A5

The pancreas should be imaged and its exocrine function assessed. Imaging modalities to consider include: abdominal radiograph (to show calcification – present in 30 per cent of cases), ultrasonography and computed tomography (CT). The latter two have similar specificities (85–90 per cent), but CT is more sensitive than ultrasonography (75 per cent vs 65 per cent). Exocrine function is currently best tested by the pancreolauryl test – which is non-invasive, cheap and easy to perform. Faecal fats are no longer routinely available.

 Q6: What other issues should be addressed?

A6

After confirming the diagnosis, the diet should be modified – fats can be eaten and should not be avoided because the patient will continue to lose weight. However, adequate pancreatic replacement therapy should be prescribed along with acid-suppressing drugs. Pancreatic enzymes are usually buffered by bicarbonate secretion; however, in chronic pancreatitis there may be too little bicarbonate so acid suppression is essential.

 CASE 8.5 – A 26-year-old woman with abdominal pain and vomiting.

 Q1: What specific questions would you ask the patient?

A1

Earlier episodes of right upper quadrant pain suggest biliary colic. The episode accompanied by jaundice and dark urine suggests that a stone may have obstructed the common bile duct. The present problem suggests acute gallstone pancreatitis. As with any abdominal pain, the site, radiation, and exacerbating and relieving factors should be sought. Acute pancreatitis should always be considered in patients with acute abdominal pain.

 Q2: What is the most likely diagnosis?

A2

The most likely diagnosis is acute pancreatitis. The differential diagnosis for its aetiology is gallstone pancreatitis, hereditary hypertriglyceridaemia and drug-induced pancreatitis. The differential diagnosis of the pain is cholecystitis, peptic ulcer disease (≡ perforation) and Crohn's disease.

 Q3: What examination would you perform?

A3

A full physical examination is necessary with particular attention being paid to the abdomen. Signs range from epigastric tenderness to a full-blown acute abdomen with distension and rigidity. The Grey–Turner and Cullen signs should be sought. An epigastric mass (pseudocyst) may be present. Shock may also be present.

Q4: What would be the initial management?

A4

The first step in the management is to confirm the clinical diagnosis. Blood samples should be taken for amylase, calcium, glucose and 'blood gases'. Amylase is elevated threefold in most cases of acute pancreatitis; however, occasionally very shocked patients have a normal amylase. Acidosis, hyperglycaemia and hypocalcaemia are all poor prognostic indicators. The patient should receive analgesia (pethidine), an antiemetic, resuscitation with oxygen and intravenous fluids. Hyperglycaemia should be corrected with an insulin infusion. Early senior review of patients who are shocked or have other poor prognostic indicators is imperative.

 Q5: What investigations would you request to confirm a diagnosis?

A5

The pancreas should be imaged. Imaging modalities to consider include abdominal radiograph (to exclude a perforated viscus and possibly to show a sentinel loop). Ultrasonography and CT are preferable. Ultrasonography is useful because it can show gallstones as well as pancreatic necrosis; however, bowel gas may obscure the view. Computed tomography is more accurate than ultrasonography for grading the pancreatic damage (90 per cent versus 73 per cent). Endoscopic retrograde cholangiopancreatography (ERCP) has a role – primarily to treat the underlying pathology. Without intervention, 30–50 per cent of patients with gallstone pancreatitis have further episodes.

 Q6: What other issues should be addressed?

A6

After confirming the diagnosis, the patient should undergo supportive therapy. An underlying cause should be sought. ERCP is recommended.

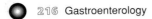 **CASE 8.6 – A 48-year-old man with alcohol problems with chronic abdominal pain.**

Q1: What specific questions would you ask the patient?

A1

Epigastric pain may arise from pathology in three main sites: stomach/duodenum, gallbladder and pancreas. An accurate description of the pain may help differentiate biliary colic from pancreatic and gastroduodenal pain – the latter two are not colicky. Pancreatic pain tends to last for days or weeks rather than hours, as in the case of peptic ulceration. The relationship to food and lack of relief with antacids, etc, should be sought.

Q2: What is the most likely diagnosis?

A2

The most likely diagnosis is alcoholic chronic pancreatitis. Patients' pain often precedes exocrine failure in people with alcohol problems.

 Q3: What examination would you perform?

A3

A full physical examination is necessary with particular attention being paid to the abdomen and the nutritional status.

 Q4: What would be the initial management?

A4

The first step in the management is to confirm the clinical diagnosis. This can be problematic in the absence of exo- and endocrine failure. The diagnosis is largely clinical, supported by anatomical changes when the pancreas is imaged and in the absence of other pathology such as duodenal ulcer disease.

 Q5: What investigations would you request to confirm a diagnosis?

A5

The pancreas should be imaged. Imaging modalities to consider include: abdominal radiograph (to show calcification – present in 30 per cent of cases), ultrasonography and CT. The latter have similar specificities (85–90 per cent), although CT is more sensitive than ultrasonography (75 versus 65 per cent). Exocrine failure is not clinically apparent until 90 per cent of the exocrine function has been lost. It is currently best tested by the Pancreolauryl test – which is non-invasive, cheap and easy to perform. Faecal fats are no longer routinely available.

 Q6: What other issues should be addressed?

A6

After confirming the diagnosis, the patient should receive pain relief in line with the World Health Organization's (WHO's) 'pain ladder'. Most patients require opiates and these should not be withheld because of concerns about their long-term use. Of patients, 50 per cent respond to a nerve block. Surgery is seldom indicated.

👥 OSCE Counselling Cases – Answers

OSCE COUNSELLING CASE 8.3 – 'Why have I got pancreatitis?'

The answer is: 'Unfortunately, your pancreas has become inflamed, this is called pancreatitis. The pancreas is an organ that lies besides the gallbladder. Stones have grown in your gallbladder. One (or some) of these stones has passed into the tube that links the gallbladder to the intestine. In this site, the same tube joins to the pancreas. As a result of the stone lying in these tubes, the pancreas has become inflamed. Pancreatitis may also be caused by alcohol and drugs: there is no suggestion that this is the case for you.'

This is an important test of communication skills. The key is to explain the anatomy of the biliary tree and how the gallstones lead to pancreatitis.

It is important to explain that pancreatitis is a result of gallstones. As it can be a result of alcohol abuse, the patient should be reassured that you understand that her pancreatitis is not so caused. The explanation of diseases that may, or may not, be confused with those that are associated with social stigma require particular skill and tact.

Be prepared to discuss the management of any condition, the nature of which you have been asked to explain.

OSCE COUNSELLING CASE 8.4 – 'Why should I stop drinking?'

The answer is 'Your drinking has led to a serious disorder of your pancreas. This disorder may cause severe abdominal pain and failure to digest your food (resulting in weight loss); if severe you may need surgery. In some patients it can be fatal. As alcohol is the cause, it is important that you stop drinking in order to reduce of the risk of further severe attacks. If you continue to drink the problem is likely to get worse. If you stop, the disease may not progress.'

In answering this question it is crucial to be both honest and understanding.

Patients may continue to have pain even if they do stop drinking. There is no place for blaming the patient if the pain continues. Supportive measures should be offered.

Additional means of controlling the pain are likely to be called for including long-term analgesics, nerve blocks and even surgery.

INFLAMMATORY BOWEL DISEASE

? Questions for each of the clinical case scenarios given

Q1: What specific questions would you ask the patient?
Q2: What is the most likely diagnosis?
Q3: What examination would you perform?
Q4: What would be the initial management?
Q5: What investigations would you request to confirm a diagnosis?
Q6: What other issues should be addressed?

Clinical cases

● CASE 8.7 – A 20-year old woman with ulcerative colitis.

A 20-year-old woman with ulcerative colitis has had symptoms for several weeks so she presents to the accident and emergency department (A&E).

● CASE 8.8 – An 18-year-old man with colicky, central, abdominal pain and vomiting after meals.

An 18-year-old male smoker presents with colicky, central, abdominal pain and vomiting 30–60 min after meals. He had been told that he may have IBD, but his mother is concerned because he has lost weight.

● CASE 8.9 – A 21-year-old man with diarrhoea and a perianal abscess.

He has noted episodes of colicky lower abdominal pain over several months and it had been suggested that he may have IBD.

👥 OSCE Counselling Cases

OSCE COUNSELLING CASE 8.5 – 'Will I get cancer?'

A 36-year-old man with established ulcerative colitis has heard that there is a risk of bowel cancer in patients with the condition. He asks: 'Will I get cancer?'

OSCE COUNSELLING CASE 8.6 – 'Will I need to have the bag?'

A 20-year-woman old with refractory ulcerative colitis is concerned that surgery is imminent. She asks: 'Will I need to have the bag?'

🔑 Key concepts

In order to work through the core clinical cases in this chapter, you will need to understand the following key concepts.

Patients with IBD often present with symptoms that have been present for several weeks or months. Many will have been told that they have IBS.

A history and examination will often point to the correct diagnosis by the time such patients present.

Patients should be counselled about the need for potentially embarrassing invasive investigations and the probable long-term nature of IBD, and encouraged to seek help from reputable sources such as the National Association for Colitis and Crohn's Disease (NACC).

Answers

 CASE 8.7 – A 20-year old woman with ulcerative colitis.

 Q1: What specific questions would you ask the patient?

A1

The severity of the attack should be assessed. Specifically, the frequency and consistency of the stool should be assessed. The presence of blood should be sought. The presence, periodicity and site of abdominal pain should be assessed, as should any weight loss.

 Q2: What is the most likely diagnosis?

A2

Acute severe ulcerative colitis. The assessment of severity is based upon clinical observation. The differential diagnosis is infectious diarrhoea and hypersensitivity to her treatment.

 Q3: What examination would you perform?

A3

A full physical examination is necessary with particular attention being paid to the signs of disease severity (fever, anaemia, tachycardia) and to abdominal signs. Fever, anaemia and tachycardia define severe disease.

 Q4: What would be the initial management?

A4

The first step in the management is to corroborate the clinical diagnosis. Blood samples should be taken for FBC, C-reactive protein (CRP) and albumin. A plain abdominal radiograph should be performed to assess colonic diameter as well as to look for mucosal islands. Stool cultures should be performed. The patient should be admitted, commenced on intravenous hydrocortisone 100 mg four times daily and heparin 5000 U s.c. three times daily. A stool chart should be commenced, recording the frequency and amount of stool, and the presence of blood. Weight should be recorded.

 Q5: What investigations would you request to confirm a diagnosis?

A5

Senior review should be sought with a view to considering a cautious, limited sigmoidoscopy. Sigmoidoscopy is potentially dangerous.

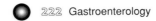

 Q6: What other issues should be addressed?

A6

If after 3–5 days the CRP and stool frequency have not improved, a surgical opinion should be sought with a view to colectomy on day 7. Some centres recommend abdominal radiograph on alternate days. A deterioration in the abdominal radiograph or the physical signs should prompt earlier surgical review.

● **CASE 8.8 – An 18-year-old man with colicky, central, abdominal pain and vomiting after meals.**

 Q1: What specific questions would you ask the patient?

A1

The pain should be assessed, looking for site, radiation, and exacerbating and relieving factors, as well as special precipitating factors – particularly foods. The frequency of the vomiting and its relationship to the pain (and meals) should be clarified. The amount of weight lost should be documented and the duration of this symptom. A family and travel history should be taken. Medication should be recorded.

 Q2: What is the most likely diagnosis?

A2

The symptoms suggest subacute obstruction. The differential diagnoses include adhesions, Crohn's disease and intussusception.

 Q3: What examination would you perform?

A3

A full physical examination is necessary with particular attention being paid to the nutritional state, signs of inflammatory disease (fever, anaemia, tachycardia) and abdominal signs – specifically looking for a mass.

 Q4: What would be the initial management?

A4

The patient may warrant admission if he is malnourished, dehydrated or in pain. However, subacute obstruction is often investigated as an outpatient. If admitted he will need: analgesia, intravenous fluid replacement (2–3 L/day) and a nasogastric tube (to decompress the upper GI tract). Initial investigation of the admitted patient should include: abdominal radiograph (for obstruction), U&Es, LFTs and FBC with CRP and plasma viscosity (PV). If not admitted, investigate as in the answer below.

Q5: What investigations would you request to confirm a diagnosis?

A5

After resuscitation (or in the outpatient setting), urgent barium follow-through (or small bowel enema) should be performed. CT and/or ultrasonography may be indicated if there is a mass. CT will show the 'pseudo-kidney sign' if intussusception is present.

 Q6: What other issues should be addressed?

A6

Subacute obstruction may be managed conservatively while the diagnosis is reached. Most cases come to surgery in the long term.

 CASE 8.9 – A 21-year-old man with diarrhoea and a perianal abscess.

 Q1: What specific questions would you ask the patient?

A1

The diarrhoea should be assessed with regard to: frequency, duration, the presence of blood and mucus, and its relationship to the abdominal pain. Constitutional symptoms – fever, and weight loss – should also be sought. With regard to his abscess, duration of symptoms, and the site and radiation of the pain should be determined. Previous episodes and their treatment should be recorded. Lifestyle, travel and a family history should be noted.

 Q2: What is the most likely diagnosis?

A2

The most likely diagnosis is Crohn's disease. Diarrhoea need not be accompanied by blood in patients with Crohn's disease. Perianal abscess may accompany ulcerative colitis.

 Q3: What examination would you perform?

A3

A full physical examination is necessary with particular attention being paid to the abdomen, nutritional status, evidence of systemic illness (fever, tachycardia, anaemia) and the perineum. Per rectal examination is not indicated because the abscess encroaches on the anus. An examination under anaesthetic is preferred.

Q4: What would be the initial management?

A4

The first steps in the management are to relieve suffering and confirm the clinical diagnosis. Pain should be relieved by analgesia while a prompt surgical opinion is sought. Investigations to support the diagnosis should be performed with FBC, LFTs, CRP and PV as a prelude to a surgical review.

 Q5: What investigations would you request to confirm a diagnosis?

A5

Generally, an examination under anaesthetic is the preferred approach to such patients. During this procedure, the abscess may be drained, a sigmoidoscopy and rectal biopsy performed, and probing performed for a fistula. A stent may be placed if the fistula is found.

Q6: What other issues should be addressed?

A6

After managing the abscess, the diagnosis of Crohn's disease should be confirmed. Imaging options include: magnetic resonance imaging (MRI) and CT. MRI is the investigation of choice for imaging the soft tissues around the rectum and demonstrating fistulas which usually underlie abscesses in Crohn's disease. Crohn's disease should be managed by draining the abscess, seeking out and treating other foci of infection, and treating the disease itself.

👥 OSCE Counselling Cases – Answers

OSCE COUNSELLING CASE 8.5 – 'Will I get cancer?'

The answer is 'There is an increased risk of bowel cancer in some patients with ulcerative colitis. This risk does not apply to all patients. Young patients with extensive disease that has a grumbling course seem to be at greatest risk. The medication that is given for the treatment of colitis (mesalazine) appears to lower the risk of bowel cancer. We will assess your risk by plotting your disease extent. If the risk appears to be increased, we will discuss measures that may enable us to detect it at an early stage. Although the risk to patients with ulcerative colitis of getting bowel cancer is greater than that of people without colitis, the risk to an individual patient remains relatively small.'

It is important to be honest, but to offer reassurance at the same time.

Relative risk and absolute risk may be difficult concepts to explain to patients. It is worth planning your answer to such common questions.

OSCE COUNSELLING CASE 8.6 – 'Will I need to have the bag?'

The answer is 'Yes, at least in the short term'. Patients with refractory disease are often taking steroids at the time of surgery and so the surgery is kept as simple as possible. The operation of choice is to remove as much diseased bowel as possible without operating deep in the pelvis. (A subtotal colectomy, oversewing the rectum above the levators.) A stoma will be necessary. Most patients feel better very quickly and many soon adapt to the stoma. These patients will later need a second operation to remove the rectum (a proctectomy). Other patients may prefer an ileoanal pouch. The pouch brings about improved body image, but is associated with the need to pass stool frequently (typically four to six times a day). Of patients, 15–20 per cent lose their bowel (undergo colectomy) in the long term.

It is important to differentiate the emergency situation in which the priority is to keep the patient alive and healthy, from the elective situation where the aim is to restore quality of life.

Ileoanal pouches are not a panacea. The quality of life of patients with a pouch is only as good as that in patients with mild ulcerative colitis. The stool of a patient with a pouch is likely to be loose and passed frequently.

Pouchitis with bloody looser stools occurs in 5–20 per cent of patients. It can often be managed medically, but may result in a reversal of the pouch and recreation of the stoma.

PEPTIC ULCER DISEASE

Q1: What is the likely differential diagnosis?
Q2: What in the given history supports the diagnosis?
Q3: What additional features in the history would you seek to support a particular diagnosis?
Q4: What clinical examination would you perform and why?
Q5: What investigations would be most helpful and why?
Q6: What treatment options are appropriate?

Clinical cases

● CASE 8.10 – 'Doctor, I have indigestion.'

A 70-year-old man with arthritis and ischaemic heart disease presents with indigestion. He has epigastric pain radiating to his back. He has been taking aspirin for his heart and ibuprofen for his arthritis.

● CASE 8.11 – 'Doctor, I have indigestion and cannot eat properly.'

A 35-year-old woman presents with a feeling of discomfort after eating meals. She describes a fullness after eating a modest amount, and can no longer finish the meal that she used to eat. The indigestion is also troublesome.

● CASE 8.12 – 'Doctor, I am worried that I am losing weight and vomiting.'

A 60-year-old man is brought to see you accompanied by his wife. Together they describe that he has had progressively worsening vomiting for some months. He has lost a stone in weight. He finds that the vomiting is worse after a full meal, but liquids trouble him less than solid food. In the past he has suffered from indigestion and has taken over-the-counter remedies for this.

▇▇ OSCE Counselling Cases

OSCE COUNSELLING CASE 8.7 – 'Can I take aspirin for my heart now that I have an ulcer?'

OSCE COUNSELLING CASE 8.8 – 'The tablets for my ulcer were wonderful. Should I continue to take them?'

🔑 Key concepts

In order to work through the core clinical cases in this chapter, you will need to understand the following key concepts.

What is the aetiology of peptic ulcers?

Helicobacter pylori is found in > 90 per cent of patients with duodenal ulcers and 70 per cent of patients with gastric ulcers. NSAIDs contribute to the aetiology of peptic ulcer disease. Smoking and alcohol are minor contributory factors.

How are they diagnosed?

The gold standard is the demonstration of an ulcer by endoscopy or barium meal. Endoscopy is preferable because gastric ulcers can be biopsied, to look for malignancy, and *H. pylori* can be sought in the stomach of patients with peptic ulcers, whether gastric or duodenal.

How are they treated?

As most ulcers are *H. pylori* related, *H. pylori* eradication should be prescribed. This consists of a PPI and two antibiotics from metronidazole, amoxicillin and clarithromycin.

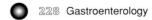
Answers

 CASE 8.10 – 'Doctor, I have indigestion.'

 Q1: What is the likely differential diagnosis?

A1

- Peptic ulcer disease
- Carcinoma of the stomach
- Carcinoma of the pancreas.

 Q2: What in the given history supports the diagnosis?

A2

Indigestion-like symptoms are usually a result of gastroduodenal disease. The diseases include mucosal inflammation (gastritis, duodenitis) and ulceration. Most duodenal ulcer disease is associated with *H. pylori*; NSAIDs, including aspirin and ibuprofen, enhance the risk of ulcer disease occurring in patients without *H. pylori* infection. This man is of an age where ulcer-complicating *H. pylori* is quite common. His consumption of NSAIDs increases his risk.

 Q3: What additional features in the history would you seek to support a particular diagnosis?

A3

It is important to ask the patient about weight loss, because this may indicate that the patient has a carcinoma. His NSAID medication should be reviewed. Evidence from his history of earlier ulcer symptoms before the current episode should be sought.

Q4: What clinical examination would you perform and why?

A4

Full physical examination should be performed with particular attention paid to lymphadenopathy in the neck, which might indicate metastatic disease from carcinoma of the stomach. The epigastrium should be examined with particular care for a mass. The liver edge should be identified. An irregular edge might indicate a carcinoma.

Q5: What investigations would be most helpful and why?

A5

An endoscopy (oesophagogastroduodenoscopy) should be performed to look for peptic ulcer disease and to rule out carcinoma of the stomach. Histology should be obtained for *H. pylori*.

 Q6: What treatment options are appropriate?

A6

If the patient has *H. pylori* triple therapy should be prescribed followed by a long-term PPI to protect him against future non-NSAID-associated risks. If he is *H. pylori* negative PPI drugs should be used alone. If the patient is found to have carcinoma of the stomach, it should be staged and surgery considered. Patients with a gastric ulcer should undergo repeat endoscopy after 6 weeks to ensure healing and to facilitate repeat biopsy to obtain further histological samples.

● CASE 8.11 – 'Doctor, I have indigestion and cannot eat properly.'

 Q1: What is the likely differential diagnosis?

A1

Differential diagnosis is non-ulcer dyspepsia and peptic ulcer disease. Gastric cancer is very unlikely in a patient of this age. The role of *H. pylori* in the absence of ulceration in such patients is not clear.

Early satiety (feeling fullness before completing a meal) is associated with non-ulcer dyspepsia. However, it may also occur in patients with gastric outlet obstruction and carcinoma of the stomach. The patient's age make these considerations unlikely.

 Q2: What in the given history supports the diagnosis?

A2

Non-ulcer dyspepsia is a functional disorder often exacerbated by stress. Stressors should be investigated. The early satiety means that non-ulcer dyspepsia is the most likely explanation although, if vomiting is present, carcinoma of the stomach and/or other sinister pathology should be considered.

 Q3: What additional features in the history would you seek to support a particular diagnosis?

A3

It is important, in the history, to look for the patient's ethnic background and family history, either of which might increase the risk of peptic ulcer disease. Exposure to NSAIDs should be sought in the history – these may be over-the-counter remedies. Consumption of alcohol and cigarettes should be investigated, although these are small contributory factors to peptic ulcer disease compared with *H. pylori*.

Q4: What clinical examination would you perform and why?

A4

Full examination should be performed with consideration given to lymphadenopathy and epigastric mass. Such features are not expected in patients with non-ulcer dyspepsia.

 Q5: What investigations would be most helpful and why?

A5

It is useful to look for *H. pylori* in young patients with dyspepsia. There are several ways in which this can be conducted. *H. pylori* can be identified by a urease breath test, necessitating a trip to the local hospital. *H. pylori* infection can be sought using serology. Most GPs can perform this test and send the sample to a reference laboratory. Finally, endoscopy might be used although, in a patient of this age, it is not usually indicated.

 Q6: What treatment options are appropriate?

A6

Triple therapy may be prescribed for the patient if *H. pylori* positive: a PPI with two antibiotics from metronidazole, amoxicillin and clarithromycin (typically one is metronidazole). It is important to stop PPI therapy after *H. pylori* has been eradicated. Domperidone may also be prescribed to aid gastric emptying by increasing its motility.

CASE 8.12 – 'Doctor, I am worried that I am losing weight and vomiting.'

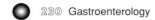 **Q1: What is the likely differential diagnosis?**

A1

- Pyloric stenosis secondary to *H. pylori*-associated peptic ulcer disease

- Carcinoma of the stomach

- Rare duodenal tumours, polyps, Crohn's disease and dysmotility syndrome.

 Q2: What in the given history supports the diagnosis?

A2

The clue to the diagnosis in this patient is previous use of over-the-counter remedies for indigestion, mainly in a patient with under-treated peptic ulcer. The vomiting suggests gastric outlet obstruction.

Q3: What additional features in the history would you seek to support a particular diagnosis?

A3

Pyloric stenosis and carcinoma of the stomach may present in a similar manner.

Duodenal Crohn's disease, polyps, etc. usually have a longer history. Dysmotility syndrome is unusual except in patients with diabetes.

 Q4: What clinical examination would you perform and why?

A4

On examination anaemia, lymphadenopathy, epigastric mass and irregular liver edge should be sought.

 Q5: What investigations would be most helpful and why?

A5

Investigation is mandatory. Endoscopy and/or barium meal should be performed urgently. Computed tomography of the upper abdomen should be considered. If these investigations are negative, gastric emptying studies should be performed.

 Q6: What treatment options are appropriate?

A6

If the patient is found to have benign peptic stricture, endoscopic balloon dilatation should be considered. Surgery is called for if balloon dilatation fails. If the patient has carcinoma staging should be performed and surgery considered. If the patient has duodenal obstruction a gastroenterostomy should be performed. If the patient has dysmotility syndrome domperidone or erythromycin should be prescribed.

⛉ OSCE Counselling Cases – Answers

OSCE COUNSELLING CASE 8.7 – 'Can I take aspirin for my heart now that I have an ulcer?'

In a patient who has a good indication for non-steroidal therapy such as coronary disease, transient ischaemic attack (TIA) or inflammatory arthritis, aspirin and/or non-steroidal therapy should be resumed after the ulcer has been treated appropriately, typically with triple therapy. PPI should be co-prescribed with the non-steroidal drugs. Consider alternative of clopidogrel, which may be safer.

OSCE COUNSELLING CASE 8.8 – 'The tablets for my ulcer were wonderful. Should I continue to take them?'

The short answer to this patient is no. He should be told that the *H. pylori* infection caused the ulcer. Eradicating infection will mean that the ulcer is unlikely to return. It is important to discontinue PPI therapy because of the problems of atrophic gastritis, achlorhydria and bacterial overgrowth.

CIRRHOSIS

Q1: What is the likely differential diagnosis?
Q2: What in the given history supports the diagnosis?
Q3: What additional features in the history would you seek to support a particular diagnosis?
Q4: What clinical examination would you perform and why?
Q5: What investigations would be most helpful and why?
Q6: What treatment options are appropriate?

Clinical cases

● CASE 8.13 – 'Doctor, I have turned yellow and my stomach is swollen.'

A retired publican presents with progressive jaundice and abdominal swelling. He drinks more than 40 units of alcohol per week. Previously he has been admitted with fever and vomiting, which he was told was caused by alcohol.

● CASE 8.14 – 'My husband has become confused.'

After several days in hospital, the patient with jaundice and ascites becomes confused, disorientated and aggressive.

● CASE 8.15 – 'Doctor, please see your patient. He is vomiting blood.'

A couple of days after showing evidence of encephalopathy, this patient with chronic liver disease has haematemesis.

👥 OSCE Counselling Cases

OSCE COUNSELLING CASE 8.9 – 'Should my husband have a transplant?'

OSCE COUNSELLING CASE 8.10 – 'Why is my husband confused?'

🔑 Key concepts

In order to work through the core clinical cases in this chapter, you will need to understand the following key concepts.

How is decompensated liver disease recognized?

Decompensation is recognized from the following:

- History: jaundice, abdominal swelling, drowsiness, GI bleeding

- Examination: jaundice, fetor, flapping tremor, ascites, oedema, impaired consciousness

- Laboratory investigations: poor synthetic function – falling albumin and prolonging clotting times.

How are bleeding varices managed?

First, by resuscitating with intravenous fluids – preferably blood products, and oxygen. Second, at endoscopy with a view to injection sclerotherapy or band ligation. Finally, by Sengstaken tube placement and/or glypressin (intravenous).

How is ascites, caused by decompensated liver disease, managed?

First, ascitic fluid should be analysed for spontaneous bacterial peritonitis (SBP). If the white cell count (WCC) is > 250/mL SBP is likely and should be treated with cephalosporins or ciprofloxacin. Second, therapy should be initiated:

- Water restriction to < 1.5 L or even < 1 L/day with salt restriction

- Spironolactone should be added starting at 50 mg with a slow increase in dose

- Therapeutic paracentesis should be considered with intravenous replacement (100 ml 20 per cent human albumin solution [HAS]) per 2–2.5 L ascites drained.

Answers

 CASE 8.13 – 'Doctor, I have turned yellow and my stomach is swollen.'

 Q1: What is the likely differential diagnosis?

A1

- Decompensated cirrhosis secondary to alcohol consumption or other causes of chronic liver disease.
- Carcinoma of the pancreas (or similar upper GI cancer with liver metastases) and peritoneal spread.

 Q2: What in the given history supports the diagnosis?

A2

This man has a high-risk profession for alcoholic liver disease. His previous admission suggests that he may have had alcoholic hepatitis. He is still drinking. The abdominal swelling is likely to be the result of ascites. Together the jaundice and ascites indicate that he has decompensated cirrhosis.

 Q3: What additional features in the history would you seek to support a particular diagnosis?

A3

In the history it should be established whether he has been told that he has cirrhosis. Look for weight gain to support the diagnosis of ascites (weight loss might indicate a malignant process). Swelling of the ankles would be common in cirrhosis at this stage. Also history should be sought of previous ulcer disease that might indicate gastric cancer. Previous bowel surgery might indicate a malignant process.

 Q4: What clinical examination would you perform and why?

A4

The signs of decompensated alcoholic liver disease should be sought, including: Dupuytren's contracture, palmar erythema, spider naevi, gynaecomastia, hepatosplenomegaly and ascites.

 Q5: What investigations would be most helpful and why?

A5

Ultrasonography of the abdomen with liver biopsy should be performed at an early stage. Paracentesis should be carried out to look for a malignant process causing the ascites. The liver investigations will include hepatitis serology, autoimmune profile, serum ferritin, α-fetoprotein, anti-trypsin and ceruloplasmin.

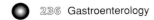 **Q6: What treatment options are appropriate?**

A6

The ascites should be treated with fluid restriction and spironolactone. If these measures do not work, paracentesis with terlipressin and albumin (HAS) cover should be instituted.

CASE 8.14 – 'My husband has become confused.'

 Q1: What is the likely differential diagnosis?

A1

Encephalopathy secondary to decompensation, sepsis, electrolyte disturbance or GI bleeding.

 Q2: What in the given history supports the diagnosis?

A2

Patients admitted with decompensated liver disease are at high risk of encephalopathy. The instrumentation for paracentesis may increase the risk of bacterial peritonitis. Venous access and urethral catheterization will increase the risk of sepsis in those sites. Treatment of ascites might precipitate encephalopathy as a result of electrolyte disturbance.

 Q3: What additional features in the history would you seek to support a particular diagnosis?

A3

From his wife and the nurses, clues should be sought for the portal of entry of infection. The nurses should be asked whether he has had haematemesis or melaena. Charts should be checked for undue diuresis.

Q4: What clinical examination would you perform and why?

A4

Full physical examination with a view to finding a focus of infection should be carried out. This must include the chest and Venflon sites, and careful abdominal palpation. Rectal examination may be necessary to rule out melaena.

Q5: What investigations would be most helpful and why?

A5

Full septic screen should be performed with paracentesis, blood cultures, chest radiograph and urine cultures.

Electrolytes should be assessed. Hb might be measured to look for evidence of sepsis (raised WCC) and anaemia (indicating GI bleed)

 Q6: What treatment options are appropriate?

A6

The most likely explanation for the deterioration is sepsis. Cephalosporins and/or ciprofloxacin should be commenced. Consideration should be given to staphylococcal infection. It will require gentamicin and/or flucloxacillin. If methicillin-resistant *Staphylococcus aureus* (MRSA) is present, vancomycin may be used. Lactulose should be started immediately. Neomycin, or more probably metronidazole, should be used to suppress bacterial growth within the bowel.

Electrolyte disturbance and hypoglycaemia should be corrected.

 CASE 8.15 – 'Doctor, please see your patient. He is vomiting blood.'

 Q1: What is the likely differential diagnosis?

A1

- Bleeding oesophageal varices
- Bleeding peptic ulcer disease.

 Q2: What in the given history supports the diagnosis?

A2

Patients with decompensated liver disease are at high risk of variceal bleeding, having demonstrated evidence of portal hypertension (through the ascites). Encephalopathy may have been precipitated by a GI bleed. Of patients with GI bleed on the background of cirrhosis, 50 per cent actually bleed from non-variceal sources.

 Q3: What additional features in the history would you seek to support a particular diagnosis?

A3

No further features could be obtained in the history of this patient.

Q4: What clinical examination would you perform and why?

A4

Evidence of GI bleeding should be assessed, including observation of melaena and assessment of BP and pulse, and sweating and anaemia should be sought.

 Q5: What investigations would be most helpful and why?

A5

Urgent endoscopy should be performed with a view to finding and treating the varices. Full blood count is likely to show anaemia, clotting tests (international normalized ratio [INR]) should be undertaken as well as a cross-match.

Q6: What treatment options are appropriate?

A6

At endoscopy (see above), banding and/or sclerotherapy should be used to stop variceal bleeding. Patients with peptic ulcer haemorrhage should receive the preferred treatment in the unit. In most hospitals this is adrenaline (epinephrine) injection.

Resuscitation with blood and/or clotting factors is mandatory. The treatment for encephalopathy should be continued and possibly increased.

👥 OSCE Counselling Cases – Answers

OSCE COUNSELLING CASE 8.9 – 'Should my husband have a transplant?'

Liver transplantation is not indicated in patients who are still drinking alcohol. The consensus of opinion is that patients should be abstinent from alcohol 6 months before surgery. In the 6 months between stopping drinking and surgery, full liver support should be offered as well as psychological assessment.

OSCE COUNSELLING CASE 8.10 – 'Why is my husband confused?'

Patients with liver disease become confused when the liver does not work properly. In this situation the risk of infection is increased and chemical upsets now occur as part of the treatment. In addition, patients with this problem can bleed internally. All of these factors lead to a disturbance of brain chemical function. However, in most patients this can be put right.

CONSTIPATION

Q1: What is the likely differential diagnosis?
Q2: What in the given history supports the diagnosis?
Q3: What additional features in the history would you seek to support a particular diagnosis?
Q4: What clinical examination would you perform and why?
Q5: What investigations would be most helpful and why?
Q6: What treatment options are appropriate?

Clinical cases

● CASE 8.16 – 'Doctor, I can't open my bowels.'

A 50-year-old man with squamous carcinoma of the bronchus and bony mestastases is referred complaining of abdominal distension. He has not opened his bowels for 8 days. His abdominal pain has worsened and he has increased his morphine sulphate tablets (MST), which previously he just took for bone pain.

● CASE 8.17 – 'Doctor, I don't feel as though I empty my bowel.'

A teenage girl presents with abdominal discomfort and a story of passing pellet-like stools. She experiences abdominal bloating before defecation and after defecation feels that she has not adequately emptied her bowels.

● CASE 8.18 – 'Doctor, please see this man with incontinence.'

A 78-year-old man with Parkinson's disease is admitted from a nursing home with faecal incontinence. Previously he had been noted to have stubborn bowels. Both he and the nurses were surprised when he began staining his clothing.

▮▮ OSCE Counselling Cases

OSCE COUNSELLING CASE 8.9 – 'Doctor, what can be done to stop my husband who needs to take pain-killers becoming constipated again?'

OSCE COUNSELLING CASE 8.10 – 'Doctor, why can't my daughter simply take senna when she has constipation?'

Key concepts

In order to work through the core clinical cases in this chapter, you will need to understand the following key concepts.

The aetiology of constipation

Constipation is a consequence of slow or interrupted transit through the intestine, in particular the large bowel. In most patients it is a result of either drugs (anticholinergic side effects or opiates) or diet. Occasionally bowel motility is impaired by hormonal or colonic neuromuscular disorders.

How is it managed?

A careful history should be obtained. Drugs causing constipation should be stopped or further drugs given to counter the side effects. Diet should be improved, by the addition of fresh fruit and vegetables.

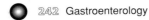

Answers

 CASE 8.16 – 'Doctor, I can't open my bowels.'

 Q1: What is the likely differential diagnosis?

A1

- Opiate-induced constipation
- Hypercalcaemia-induced constipation secondary to squamous carcinoma and/or bony metastases.

 Q2: What in the given history supports the diagnosis?

A2

Constipation is a symptom, not a disease. In this patient the risk factor for constipation is treatment with opiates. In addition, patients with bony metastases and squamous carcinoma are at risk of hypercalcaemia. This needs to be considered.

Q3: What additional features in the history would you seek to support a particular diagnosis?

A3

It is important to see whether or not the patient appears dehydrated or confused which might suggest hypercalcaemia. In the history it should also be determined whether the patient is taking laxatives while consuming MST.

Q4: What clinical examination would you perform and why?

A4

Look for evidence of dehydration that might accompany confusion, because this also indicates hypercalcaemia. This is an insidious problem and should be specifically looked for on examination. The abdomen should be palpated and a rectal examination performed

 Q5: What investigations would be most helpful and why?

A5

The main investigations will include biochemistry for hypercalcaemia and uraemia. Abdominal examination might be necessary to look for faecal loading if the patient had an empty rectum on physical examination.

Q6: What treatment options are appropriate?

A6

Most patients will respond to enemas and stimulant laxatives, e.g. senna, accompanied also by softeners such as docusate sodium. Co-danthromer is specifically indicated in patients with opiate-induced constipation in the terminal setting. If the patient has hypercalcaemia, replace fluids intravenously and consider bisphosphonate treatment.

CASE 8.17 – 'Doctor, I don't feel as though I empty my bowel.'

 Q1: What is the likely differential diagnosis?

A1

- Poor dietary habit
- Constipation-predominant irritable bowel syndrome (IBS)
- Dysmotility.
- (Myxoedema, hypercalcaemia and Hirschsprung's disease are rare causes.)

 Q2: What in the given history supports the diagnosis?

A2

This girl is a prime candidate for poor dietary intake. Girls of this age can have fickle diets. Breakfast is often avoided. The most likely explanation for her bowel disorder is poor dietary intake with an element of IBS.

 Q3: What additional features in the history would you seek to support a particular diagnosis?

A3

Full dietary history should be taken with particular attention to fruit, fibre and breakfast consumption. The history of stress should be sought, as well as a history of sexual abuse, which is more prevalent in girls with IBS than other patients. If the patient has vomiting or a family history, an underlying motility disorder might be the problem.

 Q4: What clinical examination would you perform and why?

A4

On examination look for evidence of hypothyroidism, demonstrated by dry skin and goitre, perhaps with a bradycardia. On examination of the abdomen, faecal loading should be sought. Rectal examination should be considered only after a history of sexual abuse has been sought.

Q5: What investigations would be most helpful and why?

A5

Thyroid-stimulating hormone (TSH) and calcium may be measured, but in most patients it is unnecessary. Consider transit time studies and full-thickness rectal biopsy.

 Q6: What treatment options are appropriate?

A6

Dietary advice should be given with particular reference to fruit, fibre and breakfast consumption. It might be necessary to add linseed, kiwi or other dietary laxatives to her diet. Regular medication (laxatives) should not be prescribed.

Occasionally a barium enema can be therapeutic as well as providing reassurance.

 CASE 8.18 – 'Doctor, please see this man with incontinence.'

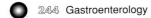 **Q1: What is the likely differential diagnosis?**

A1

- Overflow diarrhoea: secondary to medication, immobility, depression, colonic dysmotility.
- Infections including norovirus, rotavirus and *Clostridium difficile*.

 Q2: What in the given history supports the diagnosis?

A2

Parkinson's disease causes immobility, but can also cause smooth muscle dysfunction of the GI tract. Dysphagia and constipation are common. The most common cause of faecal incontinence in this kind of patient is overflow diarrhoea.

 Q3: What additional features in the history would you seek to support a particular diagnosis?

A3

It is important to look for drugs that might contribute to constipation, including traditional anticholinergic medication for Parkinson's disease. His immobility should be assessed. Patients who are bed- or chair-bound have a greater risk of constipation. Depression might also exacerbate immobility. It is not uncommon in people with Parkinson's disease. In addition, a source of infectious diarrhoea should be considered in a patient living in a nursing home.

Q4: **What clinical examination would you perform and why?**

A4

Signs of Parkinson's disease should be sought in addition to signs of faecal loading on abdominal and rectal examinations.

 Q5: **What investigations would be most helpful and why?**

A5

If the patient has a loaded colon on physical examination, no investigation is called for. If the patient has an empty rectum and no faecal loading on abdominal radiograph an infection screen should be performed.

 Q6: **What treatment options are appropriate?**

A6

An enema followed by oral laxative should be prescribed to this patient. Consideration should be given to stopping anticholinergic drugs and dealing with any depression.

👥 OSCE Counselling Cases – Answers

OSCE COUNSELLING CASE 8.9 – 'Doctor, what can be done to stop my husband who needs to take pain-killers becoming constipated again?'

Stimulant laxatives should be prescribed in all patients receiving opiate medication. The frequency and strength of the laxative should match its strength. A prescription with such laxatives should prevent further problems.

OSCE COUNSELLING CASE 8.10 – 'Doctor, why can't my daughter simply take senna when she has constipation?'

It is important to treat the cause of the constipation rather than the effect. Senna is a stimulant laxative that can lead to problems later in life if started in such young patients. It is better to have a healthy, mixed diet to help with normal GI function than to use laxatives.

HEPATITIS

? Questions for each of the clinical case scenarios given

Q1: What is the likely differential diagnosis?
Q2: What in the given history supports the diagnosis?
Q3: What additional features in the history would you seek to support a particular diagnosis?
Q4: What clinical examination would you perform and why?
Q5: What investigations would be most helpful and why?
Q6: What treatment options are appropriate?

Clinical cases

● CASE 8.19 – An 18-year-old student returning from India with jaundice.

An 18-year-old student has returned from a gap year spent in India with a short history of diarrhoea, abdominal discomfort and jaundice.

● CASE 8.20 – A 30-year-old ex-drug abuser presents with mildly abnormal LFTs.

A 30-year-old ex-drug abuser presents with feeling vaguely unwell. His GP has obtained liver function tests, but are mildly abnormal with an alanine aminotransferase (ALT) of 50 IU/L (normal range < 40 IU/L).

👥 OSCE Counselling Cases

OSCE COUNSELLING CASE 8.11 – 'Doctor, I have given up my drug habit, but have hepatitis C. Do I need to be treated?'

OSCE COUNSELLING CASE 8.12 – 'Doctor, you told me I had hepatitis A. Is there a risk that I will pass it on?'

🔑 Key concepts

In order to work through the core clinical cases in this chapter, you will need to understand the following key concepts.

Which forms of hepatitis become chronic?

Hepatitis B and C may both become chronic.

How is chronic viral hepatitis managed?

Treatment is determined by the grade and stage of liver disease (activity and fibrosis). In addition, the patient must have no ongoing lifestyle risk factors for re-infection (i.e. not using intravenous drugs) or other forms of liver disease (i.e. not alcoholic).

- Hepatitis B: combination therapy with interferon-α and lamivudine is recommended.
- Hepatitis C: combination therapy with pegylated interferon-α and ribavirin is recommended.

Answers

 CASE 8.19 – An 18-year-old student returning from India with jaundice.

 Q1: What is the likely differential diagnosis?

A1

- Hepatitis (A or B)
- Amoebic abscess, Weil's disease, side effect of medication, autoimmune hepatitis.

 Q2: What in the given history supports the diagnosis?

A2

The key to the diagnosis in this patient is the trip to India. Infectious (A) hepatitis is not uncommon in people returning from this part of the world. The pain and jaundice make a hepatobiliary problem most likely. The patient is too young to have gallstones unless she has a haemolytic disorder.

 Q3: What additional features in the history would you seek to support a particular diagnosis?

A3

In the history, attention should be paid to dark urine and pale stools, which might suggest cholestatic jaundice. If the patient has abdominal pain, its site should be elicited. It is expected that hepatobiliary pain will be epigastric and right upper quadrant in site. A history of dysentery should be sought; it might predispose the patient to amoebic liver abscess. Drugs (medical and recreational) should be considered.

 Q4: What clinical examination would you perform and why?

A4

Full examination should be performed including temperature, pulse, respiration and BP. The degree of jaundice should be elicited. Anaemia should be sought. The size and texture of the liver should be found on examination. If the diaphragm appears to be raised on the right side, consideration should be given to amoebic abscess.

Q5: What investigations would be most helpful and why?

A5

Hepatitis serology should be performed urgently (hepatitis A and B). Amoebic serology might be considered. Ultrasonography of the liver should be performed to look for an abscess. Autoimmune profile should be obtained. LFTs, FBC, INR and malaria screen should also be obtained.

Q6: What treatment options are appropriate?

A6

The treatment of hepatitis A and B is supportive. Weil's disease is treated with penicillin-based antibiotics. Liver abscess requires drainage and treatment of the underlying infection. Autoimmune hepatitis should be treated with steroids.

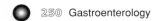 **CASE 8.20 – A 30-year-old ex-drug abuser presents with mildly abnormal LFTs.**

 Q1: What is the likely differential diagnosis?

A1

- Hepatitis C
- Non-alcoholic steatohepatitis (NASH)
- Hepatitis B.

 Q2: What in the given history supports the diagnosis?

A2

The patient's lifestyle predisposes him to hepatitis B and C, particularly hepatitis C. Modest elevation of ALT is more suggestive of hepatitis C than anything else. However, NASH can give a similar picture.

Q3: What additional features in the history would you seek to support a particular diagnosis?

A3

Look for previous jaundice in the history that would suggest hepatitis B. If the patient is obese NASH is a possibility. A history of alcohol consumption should be sought.

Q4: What clinical examination would you perform and why?

A4

On examination stigmata of chronic liver disease should be sought for patients with hepatitis. If there are no signs other than simple obesity NASH is likely.

Q5: What investigations would be most helpful and why?

A5

For hepatitis C, the investigations are serology (antibody to hepatitis C), polymerase chain reaction (PCR) for viral load, followed by liver biopsy, preferably guided by ultrasonography. The hepatitis B serology and liver biopsy are required. For NASH (hepatitis B- and C-negative patients), an ultrasonically guided liver biopsy should be obtained.

 Q6: What treatment options are appropriate?

A6

If the patient is no longer taking drugs and the liver biopsy shows viral hepatitis of sufficient stage and grade, antiviral therapy should be undertaken: interferon and either ribavirin or lamivudine for hepatitis B and C respectively. If the patient has NASH, weight reduction should be encouraged. If the patient appears to be drinking more alcohol than was apparent initially, then abstinence should be encouraged.

ᴘᴘ OSCE Counselling Cases – Answers

OSCE COUNSELLING CASE 8.11 – 'Doctor, I have given up my drug habit, but have hepatitis C. Do I need to be treated?'

Treatment for hepatitis C is determined by the stage and grade of the disease (the severity). This is determined by a liver biopsy. Any patients who have active inflammation, but no cirrhosis, are candidates for antiviral therapy. Some patients require no therapy, but need repeat biopsy instead.

OSCE COUNSELLING CASE 8.12 – 'Doctor, you told me I had hepatitis A. Is there a risk that I will pass it on?'

Hepatitis A is transmitted through poor hygiene. With good hand washing, there is no chance of passing the virus. The virus appears only in faeces and very good hygiene will prevent its transmission.

IRRITABLE BOWEL SYNDROME

? Questions for each of the clinical case scenarios given

Q1: What is the likely differential diagnosis?
Q2: What in the given history supports the diagnosis?
Q3: What additional features in the history would you seek to support a particular diagnosis?
Q4: What clinical examination would you perform and why?
Q5: What investigations would be most helpful and why?
Q6: What treatment options are appropriate?

Clinical cases

● **CASE 8.22 – Abdominal bloating.**

A 24-year-old housewife complains of abdominal bloating, which gets progressively worse during the day.

● **CASE 8.23 – After an elective period in India, a medical student returned to the UK with diarrhoea.**

The diarrhoea initially appeared to settle and then has gradually worsened over the 2 months before coming to see you.

● **CASE 8.24 – Straining to pass stool.**

A 42-year-old social worker presents with a story of straining to pass stool, passage of mucus and perhaps blood on the tissue paper.

♟♟ OSCE Counselling Cases

OSCE COUNSELLING CASE 8.13 – 'Doctor, I have severe bloating. Is it the result of food allergy?'

OSCE COUNSELLING CASE 8.14 – 'I have been told that I have IBS. Should I take a fibre supplement?'

Key concepts

In order to work through the core clinical cases in this chapter, you will need to understand the following key concepts.

The aetiology of irritable bowel syndrome

The aetiology is largely unknown. Irritable bowel syndrome falls under the umbrella of 'functional illness'. Most research points to a role for stress – sexual abuse seems particularly important. Post-infectious IBS is well recognized following 'food poisoning'. Food intolerance is rarely the explanation.

How it is diagnosed?

Clinically, based on the Manning or Rome criteria. It is NOT a diagnosis of exclusion.

How is it managed?

Stressors need to be identified and managed. Counselling may be necessary. Antidepressants are sometimes helpful. Specific drug therapy based on serotonin is not licensed at this time.

Answers

 CASE 8.22 – **Abdominal bloating.**

 Q1: What is the likely differential diagnosis?

A1

- IBS
- Bacterial overgrowth, lactose intolerance or IBD.

 Q2: What in the given history supports the diagnosis?

A2

Bacterial overgrowth, lactose intolerance and IBS can be difficult to separate from history alone. However, if the patient reports that certain foods (milk based) exacerbated symptoms and there is diarrhoea at the same time, lactose intolerance is a possibility. Bacterial overgrowth can mimic this.

If the patient experiences relief of abdominal pain with passing flatus or faeces, it is likely to be IBS, particularly if the symptoms are episodic.

Q3: What additional features in the history would you seek to support a particular diagnosis?

A3

It is important to look for duration of the illness. Irritable bowel syndrome often has insidious onset for many months before patients seek help. Weight gain is often the case, although weight loss might be a consequence of stress. Weight loss is, however, more likely to indicate organic disorder such as IBD or coeliac disease. Abdominal pain that is worse on the day that the stool form is different suggests IBS. Straining to finish defecation is often found with IBS patients, as is mucus. No blood should be present.

Q4: What clinical examination would you perform and why?

A4

On examination there should be no abnormal findings. In IBD, tenderness, abdominal mass or perianal abnormalities may be found.

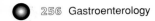 **Q5: What investigations would be most helpful and why?**

A5

No investigations are needed if a clinical diagnosis of IBS is made. However, normal CRP and plasma viscosity may be reassuring.

 Q6: What treatment options are appropriate?

A6

Irritable bowel syndrome is usually a consequence of stress. A careful social history should be obtained and attention paid to counselling around the issues described by the patient. Lactose exclusion might be helpful in some patients.

● **CASE 8.23 – After an elective period in India, a medical student returned to the UK with diarrhoea.**

 Q1: What is the likely differential diagnosis?

A1

- Post-infectious IBS
- Giardiasis.

 Q2: What in the given history supports the diagnosis?

A2

It is hard to distinguish between the differential diagnoses, but the history suggests that an infection was acquired in India, which has led to a subtle change in the bowel habit, giving chronic diarrhoea.

Q3: What additional features in the history would you seek to support a particular diagnosis?

A3

Weight loss might suggest that the patient has ongoing giardiasis. Most patients with IBS have episodic symptoms with some easing from time to time. If these symptoms do not wax and wane, it is likely that the patient has giardiasis rather than IBS.

Q4: What clinical examination would you perform and why?

A4

No abnormal findings are expected.

 Q5: What investigations would be most helpful and why?

A5

Stool culture and duodenal biopsy should be undertaken to look for *Giardia lamblia*. A therapeutic trial of metronidazole might be considered.

 Q6: What treatment options are appropriate?

A6

If the patient has giardiasis, metronidazole will cure the problem. If *Giardia lamblia* is not present it is likely that the problem is post-infectious IBS and the symptoms will gradually improve over time. Lactose avoidance may help ease the symptoms.

 CASE 8.24 – Straining to pass stool.

 Q1: What is the likely differential diagnosis?

A1

- IBS
- Mucosal prolapse
- Solitary rectal ulcer syndrome
- Gonorrhoea
- Haemorrhoids.

 Q2: What in the given history supports the diagnosis?

A2

The passage of mucus with an urge to strain suggests that the patient has rectal disease. Infrequent blood that is present only on the tissue paper makes it unlikely that the patient has proctitis. However, this is not completely ruled out.

Q3: What additional features in the history would you seek to support a particular diagnosis?

A3

It is important to determine whether there is an urge to strain at the start or the end of defecation. Both are often present in IBS. If blood is present only on days when the patient strains, this suggests that the patient has haemorrhoids or solitary rectal ulcer syndrome. Proctitis tends to give rise to frequent passage of blood in the absence of the need to strain. Sexual practice should be tactfully investigated. Anal intercourse in either sex can cause local trauma and transmit a sexually transmitted infection. Some patients self-digitate when they feel that have inadequately emptied the bowel. This can traumatize the bowel.

 Q4: What clinical examination would you perform and why?

A4

On examination nothing is expected. Sigmoidoscopy should be performed. This may show proctitis or solitary rectal ulcer in the anterior wall of the rectum. Haemorrhoids may be seen prolapsing through the anus, however protoscopy may be necessary to visualise them.

 Q5: What investigations would be most helpful and why?

A5

Flexible sigmoidoscopy should be considered. Swabs should be considered if there has been anal intercourse. Physiological studies may be necessary in patients in whom tenesmus is severe.

Q6: What treatment options are appropriate?

A6

Treatment is difficult. Stool softeners may help patients with haemorrhoids, others will require a surgical assessment with a view to band litigation or scelerotherapy. If proctitis is present it should be treated with topical therapy (steroids or 5-ASA compound). Any local infection should be treated with appropriate antibiotics or antiviral agents. However, most patients will have IBS. This may respond to hypnotherapy and, in certain situations, biofeedback; this teaches patients to respond differently to symptoms they perceive from their rectums and 'retrains' the manner in which they defecate.

♟ OSCE Counselling Cases – Answers

OSCE COUNSELLING CASE 8.13 – 'Doctor, I have severe bloating. Is it the result of food allergy?'

It is unlikely to be caused by food allergy. However, food intolerance (especially wheat) may aggravate bloating. Milk sugar (lactose) intolerance is a possibility – try avoiding all milk products (including goat's and sheep's milk) for 2 weeks and see whether this improves your symptoms.

OSCE COUNSELLING CASE 8.14 – 'I have been told that I have IBS. Should I take a fibre supplement?'

No – high-fibre diets often worsen abdominal pain in IBS. Just eat a well-balanced diet and be sure to eat a mixture of fruit and vegetables.

COELIAC DISEASE

? Questions for each of the clinical case scenarios given

Q1: What is the likely differential diagnosis?
Q2: What in the given history supports the diagnosis?
Q3: What additional features in the history would you seek to support a particular diagnosis?
Q4: What clinical examination would you perform and why?
Q5: What investigations would be most helpful and why?
Q6: What treatment options are appropriate?

Clinical cases

● CASE 8.25 – A 44-year-old woman with anaemia.

A 44-year-old woman presents with lethargy, breathlessness on exertion and a little chest tightness on walking uphill. She was turned down as a blood donor because of anaemia.

● CASE 8.26 – A 23-year-old woman presents with impaired fertility and loose stools.

She had loose stools throughout her teenage years. She is slightly built and has noted that it is difficult to increase her weight.

● CASE 8.27 – A patient with coeliac disease who infrequently attends clinic.

He presents with weight loss and anaemia at the insistence of his wife.

♟♟ OSCE Counselling Cases

OSCE COUNSELLING CASE 8.15 – 'I feel well. Why should I eat a gluten-free diet?'

OSCE COUNSELLING CASE 8.16 – 'I have coeliac disease. Are my children at risk?'

Key concepts

In order to work through the core clinical cases in this chapter, you will need to understand the following key concepts.

The aetiology of coeliac disease

Coeliac disease is a true food allergy. An immune response to the α-gliadin component of gluten leads to an immune infiltrate in the mucosa of the proximal small intestine, with secondary crypt hyperplasia and villous atrophy.

How it is diagnosed?

Antibodies to gliadin, endomysium and tissue transglutaminase are often found in the serum of patients with coeliac disease. However, these antibodies lack the sensitivity and specificity to be the gold standard for making the diagnosis. The gold standard remains the proximal small intestinal biopsy, typically obtained from the third part of the duodenum at endoscopy.

What are the complications?

Untreated coeliac disease leads to complications associated with malabsorption – anaemia (folate and iron deficiency), rickets and/or osteomalacia, bleeding disorders and subfertility.

Late complications include small bowel lymphoma and carcinomas arising in the small intestine, oesophagus, pharynx and colon.

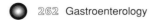

Answers

 CASE 8.25 – A 44-year-old woman with anaemia.

 Q1: What is the likely differential diagnosis?

A1

- Menorrhagia
- Dietary insufficiency (vegetarian)
- Coeliac disease.

 Q2: What in the given history supports the diagnosis?

A2

The history is consistent with progressive iron-deficiency anaemia; lack of overt blood loss in the presenting complaint suggests malabsorption or menorrhagia as likely causes.

 Q3: What additional features in the history would you seek to support a particular diagnosis?

A3

Dietary history should be obtained to exclude vegetarianism. Gynaecological history should be pursued to look for menorrhagia. A subtle change in the bowel habit should be sought that might suggest coeliac disease.

 Q4: What clinical examination would you perform and why?

A4

Nothing is expected on examination except evidence of anaemia, perhaps with cheilosis or mouth ulcers.

Q5: What investigations would be most helpful and why?

A5

Duodenal biopsy; some clinicians use anti-endomyseal antibodies as a justification for duodenal biopsy. If the dietary history is non-contributory and the gynaecological history unremarkable, coeliac disease is the most likely explanation. However, further investigations may be called for if coeliac disease is not found.

Q6: What treatment options are appropriate?

A6

Treatment of coeliac disease is a gluten-free diet with possible mineral and vitamin supplements. The patient should be encouraged to join the Coeliac Society.

 CASE 8.26 – **A 23-year-old woman presents with impaired fertility and loose stools.**

 Q1: What is the likely differential diagnosis?

A1

- Coeliac disease

- Crohn's disease

- Hormone disturbance, e.g. thyrotoxicosis

- Anorexia nervosa.

 Q2: What in the given history supports the diagnosis?

A2

The clue is the loose stool; without this the differential diagnosis would be quite broad. Anorexic patients rarely complain of inability to gain weight, so this is unlikely. Crohn's disease, thyrotoxicosis and coeliac disease are all genuine differential diagnoses of diarrhoea and subfertility.

 Q3: What additional features in the history would you seek to support a particular diagnosis?

A3

The nature of the stool should be investigated; pale, bulky, floating stools would suggest steatorrhoea; bloody diarrhoea would suggest Crohn's disease. Features of thyrotoxicosis (tremors and sweats) should be sought to rule out thyroid disease. Abdominal pain is unlikely in coeliac disease, but common in Crohn's disease.

 Q4: What clinical examination would you perform and why?

A4

On examination, little is expected in patients with coeliac disease. However, clubbing and anaemia may be present. Mouth ulcers are also relatively common. A goitre would point to thyroid dysfunction and proptosis would suggest Graves' disease.

Q5: What investigations would be most helpful and why?

A5

Anti-endomyseal antibodies and/or duodenal biopsy should be obtained. Duodenal biopsies are standard investigation. Thyroid function should be assessed if the duodenal biopsy is normal. Consideration should be given to a barium follow-through.

 Q6: What treatment options are appropriate?

A6

- The treatment for coeliac disease is a gluten-free diet.

- The treatment for thyrotoxicosis is carbimazole and/or radiotherapy with thyroxine replacement.

- Crohn's disease is treated according to symptoms; a 5-ASA compound may be used as maintenance medication.

 CASE 8.27 – A patient with coeliac disease who infrequently attends clinic.

 Q1: What is the likely differential diagnosis?

A1

Poor compliance with relapse of coeliac disease. Lymphoma or small bowel carcinoma complicating poorly controlled coeliac disease.

Q2: What in the given history supports the diagnosis?

A2

Poor clinic attendance suggests non-compliance. History from his wife would be useful to support this.

Q3: What additional features in the history would you seek to support a particular diagnosis?

A3

Diet should be reviewed, and barium follow-through and duodenal biopsy considered.

Q4: What clinical examination would you perform and why?

A4

Lymphadenopathy may be present, but often lymphoma in the GI tract does not present with lymphadenopathy.

 Q5: What investigations would be most helpful and why?

A5

Duodenal biopsy, barium follow-through and CT scan of the abdomen.

Q6: What treatment options are appropriate?

A6

- Re-introduction of gluten-free diet for coeliac disease
- Oncological assessment with radiotherapy and/or chemotherapy (? if lymphoma.)

ⅱ OSCE Counselling Cases – Answers

OSCE COUNSELLING CASE 8.15 – 'I feel well. Why should I eat a gluten-free diet?'

Most patients with coeliac disease have insidious symptoms gradually leading to presentation with diarrhoea and/or anaemia. Without control of coeliac disease, malabsorption as a consequence will occur in most patients. Untreated coeliac disease increases the risk of lymphoma and gastrointestinal malignancy.

OSCE COUNSELLING CASE 8.16 – 'I have coeliac disease. Are my children at risk?'

There is a weak association. This is not simple inheritance such as might be found in patients with haemophilia or cystic fibrosis. Although the risk to your children is small, a delay in weaning or prolonged breast-feeding is thought to be helpful. If the child fails to thrive coeliac disease should be considered.

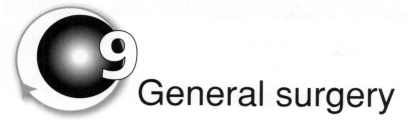

General surgery

Matthew Clark and Steven Thrush

🔑 Key concepts

Landmarks for postoperative care and complications

First 24 hours

Primary haemorrhage is the most common feature presenting as a tachycardia. Initially a fit young patient will have a stable blood pressure (BP) because the haemodynamic system is able to compensate. This is followed by hypotension because the circulatory system is no longer able to compensate. Resuscitation with colloids is essential, well before decompensation occurs.

A raised temperature (< 37.9°C) in the first 24-hour period is usually a postoperative reactive pyrexia but a rise > 38°C is suspicious of a urinary tract infection (UTI) that was pre-existing but flared up after urinary catheterization.

24–72 hours

Infection of the urinary tract, chest, surgical wound and legs must be checked for causes for pyrexia during this time period.

After abdominal surgery, a pyrexia in this time period should also raise suspicion of direct injury to the bowel that was missed during surgery and has caused peritonitis.

7–10 days

- Secondary haemorrhage caused by infection
- Thrombrosis (deep venous or pulmonary embolus)
- Fistula formation from avascular necrosis (diathermy burns) presenting as late complication, e.g. ureteric fistula, vesicovaginal fistula, rectovaginal fistula or bowel perforation causing peritonitis.

The four Bs

Decision aid for emergencies needing surgical intervention as out-of-hours procedure – remembered as the four 'B's:

Block, e.g. subacute obstruction

Bleed, e.g. peptic ulceration

Burst, e.g. ectopic pregnancy

Break, e.g. bones requiring repair.

HERNIAS

? **Questions for each of the clinical case scenarios given**

Q1: What is the likely differential diagnosis?
Q2: What issues in the given history support the diagnosis?
Q3: What additional features in the history would you seek to support a particular diagnosis?
Q4: What clinical examination would you perform and why?
Q5: What investigations would be most helpful and why?
Q6: What treatment options are appropriate?

Clinical cases

● CASE 9.1 – 'I've developed a new lump in my groin.'

A 25-year-old army sergeant suddenly develops a golfball-sized, slightly tender lump in his right groin after lifting some heavy equipment, and states that he felt a 'tearing' sensation as it happened. He is referred by the army medics to the accident and emergency department (A&E).

● CASE 9.2 – 'I can't push the lump away anymore.'

A 67-year-old retired builder presents to the outpatient clinic with a slightly tender lump in his left groin. In the past it has often disappeared overnight and was more noticeable after exertion – he had been able to 'push' the lump back inside. His health is otherwise fine, but he does cough as a result of years of smoking. Over the last 2 weeks, he has no longer been able to reduce the lump.

● CASE 9.3 – 'My hernia is sore, and I've started to vomit.'

A slim 73-year-old woman has had a groin lump for some time, which she ignored. Over the last 3 days it has become progressively more painful, with redness of the overlying skin. She has not passed a bowel motion during this time (unusual for her), and yesterday she started to vomit.

👥 OSCE Counselling Cases

OSCE COUNSELLING CASE 9.1 – 'Should I have my hernia repaired?'

A 47-year-old man presents, via his GP, with an intermittent left groin mass, causing only moderate symptoms. Examination confirms an inguinal hernia that can easily be reduced.

Q1: If an operation is offered, what specific risks should the patient be warned about?

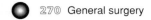

OSCE COUNSELLING CASE 9.2 – 'Why did my surgeon suggest I have my prostate 're-bored' first?'

An otherwise well 73-year-old man has a right inguinal hernia and elects to proceed with hernia repair. On history, however, he admits to slight difficulty initiating urination, poor urinary stream and nocturia (he gets up three times each night on average). The surgeon suggests a visit to a urologist before proceeding with the operation.

Q1: What factors might the surgeon be thinking about in deferring the operation?

Q2: What will the urologist do?

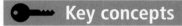

Key concepts

In order to work through the core clinical cases in this section, you will need to understand the following key concepts.

What is a hernia?

> 'A protrusion of a viscus beyond its proper cavity is denominated a hernia.'
> Sir Astley Cooper

Where do they occur?

Hernias may occur anywhere in the body. Groin hernias are the most common, usually occurring through the complex anatomy of the inguinal canal. Other sites for hernias include where musculofascial weaknesses may develop (diaphragm, lumbar triangle, edge of rectus abdominis), where abnormal stresses are found (cerebral tumours causing 'coning') or as a complication of wound healing ('incisional hernia').

What can they contain?

Just about anything. Omentum and the mobile small bowel are the usual suspects, but most organs (including the pregnant uterus) have been described in hernias at various points. Sometimes the organs may have pathology, such as Meckel's diverticulum (the rare Littre's hernia).

Why are they important?

As well as discomfort from the hernia itself, the main importance is the risk of complications. Scarring may lead to irreducibility of contents (incarceration) and possibly obstruction of any contained bowel. If the blood supply of the contents is compromised, this may cause ischaemia (strangulation), necrosis and even perforation.

Answers

 CASE 9.1 – 'I've developed a new lump in my groin.'

 Q1: What is the likely differential diagnosis?

A1

- Inguinal hernia

- Femoral hernia

- Enlarged lymph node

- Rare: saphena varix (dilatation of saphenofemoral junction); aneurysm; tumour.

 Q2: What issues in the given history support the diagnosis?

A2

Groin hernias may be caused by heavy exertion, but often no precipitating event is determined and the onset is slower. Tenderness is common, particularly in an acute-onset hernia, but may also be a feature of an inflamed lymph node. The young age of the patient makes the rarer conditions less likely.

 Q3: What additional features in the history would you seek to support a particular diagnosis?

A3

Ask whether the patient has had hernias before (making future hernias more likely) and about a family history of hernias.

 Q4: What clinical examination would you perform and why?

A4

Examine the groin and external genitalia. The diagnostic characteristic of a hernia is a cough impulse, in a mass passing through the inguinal canal (indirect inguinal hernia), sometimes right down into the scrotum, or sometimes directly through the medial posterior wall of the inguinal canal (direct inguinal hernia). Although technically possible to distinguish between indirect and direct hernias, it makes no difference to treatment.

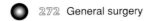 Q5: What investigations would be most helpful and why?

A5

- Ultrasonography may be useful to differentiate between clinically unclear entities.

- Fine-needle aspiration biopsy (FNAC) of enlarged lymph node(s) if detected.

 Q6: What treatment options are appropriate?

A6

- Supportive: hernia trusses have been used in the past, but play no useful role.

- Medical: no role.

- Surgical: hernia repair (herniorraphy, hernioplasty) is recommended for most patients with a groin hernia, in order to minimize the risks of future complications. The most common option for repair is an open approach through the groin (usually using a permanently implanted plastic mesh), although a laparoscopic approach is possible and may be useful for recurrent hernias, bilateral hernias and in high-performance athletes.

Ideally, the patient should stay in hospital and have his hernia repaired on the next available operating list. Realistically, he will probably be sent home for an early operation date.

CASE 9.2 – 'I can't push the lump away anymore.'

  Q1: What is the likely differential diagnosis?

A1

- Inguinal hernia

- Femoral hernia, now irreducible

- Enlarged lymph node (infection, metastatic tumour)

- Femoral artery aneurysm; saphena varix.

 Q2: What issues in the given history support the diagnosis?

A2

A groin mass that has been irreducible in the past, and is no longer so, is a very clear history diagnostically. The older age of the patient also increases the likelihood.

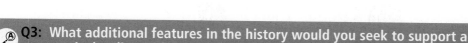

Q3: What additional features in the history would you seek to support a particular diagnosis?

A3

Ask about urinary symptoms – benign prostatic hypertropy (BPH) is not uncommon in this age group and may lead to postoperative urinary retention.

Q4: What clinical examination would you perform and why?

A4

Examine the groin and external genitalia. Carefully check the other groin for hernias; patients sometimes have a subclinical hernia on the contralateral side. Perform a digital rectal examination (DRE) to exclude prostatic enlargement.

Q5: What investigations would be most helpful and why?

A5

Ultrasonography may be useful to differentiate between clinically unclear entities.

Q6: What treatment options are appropriate?

A6

- Supportive: no role.
- Medical: no role.
- Surgical: early elective hernia repair is indicated.

CASE 9.3 – 'My hernia is sore, and I've started to vomit.'

Q1: What is the likely differential diagnosis?

A1

- Inguinal hernia, now with ischaemia and bowel obstruction
- Femoral hernia, with ischaemia and bowel obstruction
- Infected lymph node.

Q2: What issues in the given history support the diagnosis?

A2

The change in the groin lump in addition to pain, vomiting and constipation would suggest small bowel obstruction secondary to an obstructed hernia.

 Q3: What additional features in the history would you seek to support a particular diagnosis?

A3

Exclude infections that may drain to the inguinal lymph nodes. Local inflammation may explain the redness and tenderness and, if the patient is systemically unwell, this may secondarily cause paralytic ileus with vomiting.

 Q4: What clinical examination would you perform and why?

A4

Examine the groin carefully. Femoral hernia is seen more often in women than in men, although inguinal hernia is still more common. (If present, femoral hernia is more likely to cause ischaemia as a result of the tight neck of the femoral canal.) Femoral hernia will be found *below* the inguinal ligament and *medial* to the femoral arterial pulse.

 Q5: What investigations would be most helpful and why?

A5

A plain abdominal radiograph will confirm the clinical suspicion of bowel obstruction. Other investigations are directed at preparing the patient for the operating theatre.

Q6: What treatment options are appropriate?

A6

- Supportive: no role.
- Medical: bowel obstruction is associated with significant fluid and electrolyte abnormalities – the patient should be aggressively resuscitated with the expectation of going to theatre within a few hours. Nasogastric tube drainage will make the patient more comfortable, minimizing vomiting and the risk of aspiration.
- Surgical: emergency surgery is needed. This usually consists of a laparotomy (via the lower midline, although other options are available) and possibly resection of any dead bowel. Usually the ends are re-anastomosed. The hernia itself is repaired at the same time, either through the usual groin incision, or from inside the abdomen.

👥 OSCE Counselling Cases – Answers

OSCE COUNSELLING CASE 9.1 – 'Should I have my hernia repaired?'

A1

- Risks may be a result of the condition itself or the treatment of the condition.

- Risks of the treatment may be anaesthetic or operative.

- Operative risks may be those that are general to any operation or specific to this procedure.

General risks of any operation include bleeding from operative sites (minimized by careful surgery, stopping aspirin and anticoagulants if safe), wound infection (consider prophylactic antibiotics, reducing cross-contamination from other patients), early pain or discomfort.

Operative risks specific to this procedure may be early or late.

Specific risks to consider in groin hernia repair are recurrence of hernia (i.e. failure of treatment), scrotal haematoma, impairment of vascular supply to testicle (ischaemic orchitis) or late neuralgic pain from wound.

Patients usually need to make a choice about whether to proceed with an operation based on their assessment of the risks of the procedure versus the risks of the underlying condition. The best source of this information is the medical team, based on published evidence (where present) or best opinions. There is a strong consensus that groin hernia should usually be repaired surgically when present.

OSCE COUNSELLING CASE 9.2 – 'Why did my surgeon suggest I have my prostate 're-bored' first?'

A1

Benign prostatic hypertrophy is a relatively common condition in elderly men. Rarely, similar symptoms are caused by carcinoma of the prostate. Most patients cope well with their symptoms, which are usually gradual in onset. Occasionally, hernia operations may trigger acute urinary retention as a result of a combination of anaesthetic drugs, the fluid load given perioperatively and discomfort from the wound. This might require treatment with an indwelling urinary catheter; it could result in a prolonged hospital stay and perhaps leaving the catheter in place until urological assessment.

A2

A urologist will take a thorough history, perform a complete physical examination including digital rectal assessment of the prostate and arrange further investigations. The last may include blood tests for prostate-specific antigen (PSA), transrectal ultrasonography (TRUS) of the prostate, possibly with transrectal biopsy of the prostate, or cystoscopy to assess the bladder and prostatic urethra. Medications may be all that is required to minimize symptoms. Transurethral resection of the prostate (TURP) via a cystoscope may be appropriate to decrease the resistance to urinary flow; all else being equal, this is best performed before other surgery such as hernia repair.

GALLSTONES

? **Questions for each of the clinical case scenarios given**

Q1: What is the likely differential diagnosis?
Q2: What issues in the given history support the diagnosis?
Q3: What additional features in the history would you seek to support a particular diagnosis?
Q4: What clinical examination would you perform and why?
Q5: What investigations would be most helpful and why?
Q6: What treatment options are appropriate?

Clinical cases

● CASE 9.4 – 'My GP tells me my pain is caused by gallstones.'

Right upper quadrant pain after fatty meals prompts a 26-year-old woman to see her GP. The pain is felt under the ribs and in her back, and comes on over a 1-hour period, lasting up to 4 hours. It is quite severe. She is nauseated, but never vomits. The GP refers her for a surgical opinion, but suggests that the pain will probably turn out to be gallstones.

● CASE 9.5 – 'The worst ever! It's not going away, and I've got a fever.'

A 31-year-old woman has had typical biliary pain for many months, but has been reluctant to consider an operation. She now has an episode of pain that has lasted 18 hours without let-up, which she says is 'the worst ever!'. She feels flushed and has a temperature of 37.9°C. Nausea and, more recently, vomiting are a feature.

● CASE 9.6 – 'My eyes are going yellow, and my skin is itching.'

This 61-year-man has had niggling epigastric pain for some months. Over the last week his wife has commented that his eyes are yellow tinged; he has noticed that he is getting very itchy skin.

👥 OSCE Counselling Cases

OSCE COUNSELLING CASE 9.3 – 'But I don't have pain – do I need an operation?'

During an antenatal scan, a 26-year-old woman is noted to have small mobile gallstones. When questioned, she has no pain that is typical of biliary colic. She is referred by her obstetrician for a surgical opinion as to whether she should undergo cholecystectomy.

Q1: Should she be offered an operation?

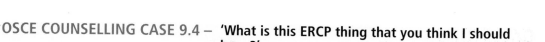

OSCE COUNSELLING CASE 9.4 – 'What is this ERCP thing that you think I should have?'

Six weeks after delivery, the same young woman develops epigastric pain and jaundice; ultrasonography reconfirms the gallstones and shows dilatation of the common bile duct to 11 mm. Endoscopic retrograde cholangiopancreatography is recommended.

Key concepts

In order to work through the core clinical cases in this chapter, you will need to understand the following key concepts.

How do gallstones form?

Bile consists of water, electrolytes, cholesterol, bile salts and lecithin (among other things). In the usual situation these are all in solution. In some patients the bile becomes 'lithogenic' (stone forming) and the constituents precipitate out around a nucleus of cellular debris or bacteria. Gallstones are formed.

What clinical problems might they cause?

Consider the problems by site:

- Gallbladder: asymptomatic, biliary pain (colic), inflammation (cholecystitis), perforation, gallbladder carcinoma
- Bile ducts: asymptomatic, obstructive jaundice, ascending cholangitis, gallstone pancreatitis
- Unusual: cholecystoenteric fistula with gallstone ileus.

What imaging options are used for gallstones and the biliary tract?

Ultrasonography is usually the investigation of choice for suspected gallstones. Plain films may show the 10 per cent of gallstones that contain calcium; HIDA scan is now mainly of historic interest. Endoscopic retrograde cholangiopancreatography gives excellent images of the lumen of the bile ducts, and allows therapeutic options such as sphincterotomy and stone extraction. Magnetic resonance cholangiopancreatography (MRCP) equals the image quality of ERCP but without the risks.

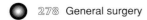
Answers

 ● CASE 9.4 – 'My GP tells me my pain is caused by gallstones.'

 Q1: What is the likely differential diagnosis?

A1

● Biliary colic

● Peptic ulcer disease.

 Q2: What issues in the given history support the diagnosis?

A2

Pain associated with gallstones commonly occurs after fatty meals, as the cholecystokin released causes the gallbladder to contract onto the stones. As a result of the hormonal nature of the stimulus, the onset is slow but the duration somewhat prolonged. Nausea is common. Back (or sometimes right shoulder) discomfort is probably the result of referred pain pathways.

Q3: What additional features in the history would you seek to support a particular diagnosis?

A3

Sometimes a family history is present, but may be a result of learned eating patterns rather than a genetic tendency to form gallstones. Check for symptoms of upper gastrointestinal (GI) bleeding or gastro-oesophageal reflux – such diseases may coexist with gallstones, making determination of whether the gallstones are truly symptomatic a challenge.

Q4: What clinical examination would you perform and why?

A4

Abdominal examination should be done, but frequently no signs are found. Check for signs of jaundice. Are there any abdominal scars? This may make a laparoscopic approach to the gallbladder more difficult.

Q5: What investigations would be most helpful and why?

A5

● Blood tests, specifically looking for evidence of ductal calculi (i.e. elevated bilirubin, amylase).

● Imaging: ultrasonography will usually show the presence of gallstones and verify that the common bile is not dilated.

Q6: What treatment options are appropriate?

A6

- Supportive: dietary modification may be tried in those who are reluctant to consider surgery. Cutting out fatty meals may reduce feelings of nausea or decrease frequency of painful episodes.
- Medical: although medical options to dissolve gallstones have been tried in the past, these are generally unsuccessful.
- Surgical: most patients with symptomatic gallstones should have the gallbladder removed (cholecystectomy). Laparoscopic cholecystectomy can be performed in around 95 per cent of patients; the remaining 5 per cent have an intraoperative conversion to an open technique or a preoperative decision to start the operation open. In some countries where laparoscopic resources are unavailable, 'mini-cholecystectomy' may result in a 5 cm scar, comparable to the total incision length of the laparoscopic approach.

● CASE 9.5 – 'The worst ever! It's not going away, and I've got a fever.'

 Q1: What is the likely differential diagnosis?

A1

- Acute cholecystitis
- Ascending cholangitis
- Right lower lobe pneumonia.

 Q2: What issues in the given history support the diagnosis?

A2

The constant nature of the pain, together with systemic unwellness, suggests supervening infection of the gallbladder.

 Q3: What additional features in the history would you seek to support a particular diagnosis?

A3

Exclude symptoms of other infections – cough, urinary frequency. If jaundice is present, ascending cholangitis (blockage by stone in common bile duct, infection ascending into liver) should be considered.

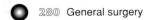

 Q4: What clinical examination would you perform and why?

A4

There may be tenderness or even peritonism in the right upper quadrant. Seek Murphy's sign – the cessation of inspiration as an inflamed gallbladder descends onto the examining fingers in the right upper quadrant. Charcot's triad (jaundice, fever, bed-shaking rigors) indicates a late stage of cholangitis.

 Q5: What investigations would be most helpful and why?

A5

Blood tests will usually show an elevated white cell count (WCC) ($> 15 \times 10^9$/L). Electrolytes should be normal unless dehydration from vomiting is present. Liver function tests (LFTs) may be mildly deranged, but high bilirubin or amylase suggests complications.

Ultrasonography will confirm stones (if not already known), and may show typical features of acute cholecystitis – wall thickening, pericholecystic fluid, the so-called 'sonographic' Murphy's sign. If perforation or abscess has occurred, these should be evident. In a severely ill patient, CT may be more appropriate.

 Q6: What treatment options are appropriate?

A6

- Supportive: fluid resuscitation and analgesia, including non-steroidal anti-inflammatory drugs (NSAIDs).
- Medical: antibiotics have traditionally been used to resolve acute cholecystitis; not all have good bile penetration so choose carefully according to local sensitivities. Often a prolonged course (10–14 days) is required. A minority fail to settle and will need operative management. Some surgeons advocate early laparoscopic cholecystectomy, claiming that it is safe and cost-effective. The alternative is a further admission in 6 weeks for elective cholecystectomy.
- Other: in a patient who is at high risk of complications, percutaneous image-guided drainage of an empyema (pus-filled gallbladder) may be considered, usually together with antibiotics.

● CASE 9.6 – 'My eyes are going yellow, and my skin is itching.'

 Q1: What is the likely differential diagnosis?

A1

- Obstructive jaundice from gallstones
- Obstructive jaundice form malignancy (e.g. pancreatic carcinoma)
- Other cause of jaundice.

Q2: What issues in the given history support the diagnosis?

A2

Pain from gallstones in the ductal system is often intermittent and difficult to characterize. Obstructive jaundice classically results in skin and scleral colour changes, and intense itch, with darker urine – all caused by bilirubin. Weight loss is a danger sign of malignancy, often indicating advanced disease.

 Q3: What additional features in the history would you seek to support a particular diagnosis?

A3

- Exclude other causes of jaundice: pre-hepatic and hepatic (compare post-hepatic or obstructive)
- Any new medications?
- Blood transfusions?
- Sickle-cell disease?

 Q4: What clinical examination would you perform and why?

A4

Carefully examine the abdomen, particularly for masses. Check the supraclavicular fossa on the left. Look for systemic signs of liver disease, starting at the hands and working centrally.

 Q5: What investigations would be most helpful and why?

A5

Blood tests should check the LFTs, including clotting parameters (which are a good overall test of hepatic synthetic function).

Imaging should start with ultrasonography, which is best for detecting the presence of gallstones. Computed tomography (CT) or magnetic resonance imaging (MRI) is superb at defining the site and characteristics of a mass, if present. ERCP and MRCP will both image the bile ducts well, but ERCP has therapeutic potential as well.

 Q6: What treatment options are appropriate?

A6

- Supportive: good hydration is important, because those with jaundice are more prone to renal impairment.
- Medical: bile-penetrating antibiotics are often started to minimize the risk of ascending infection.

- Other: ERCP with endoscopic clearance of stones is usually carried out before definitive treatment. This is not totally without risk: a small number can get pancreatitis, bleeding or perforation, or die from the procedure.

Definitive treatment involves removing the gallstone-producing factory, the gallbladder. The bile ducts can be explored intraoperatively by radiological means using an image intensifier (cholangiography) or with flexible fibreoptic instruments (choledochoscopy).

👥 OSCE Counselling Cases – Answers

OSCE COUNSELLING CASE 9.3 – 'But I don't have pain – do I need an operation?'

A1

Gallstones are common, and becoming more so with 'westernized' diets. Only about 30 per cent of those with gallstones eventually come to surgery, and generally symptoms become gradually (rather than rapidly) worse; about 2 per cent with asymptomatic gallstones develop biliary colic each year.

Some groups should have cholecystectomy considered even for asymptomatic gallstones, including those with diabetes (who have high rates of complications if cholecystitis occurs) and those with a calcified gallbladder on radiograph (associated with gallbladder cancer).

OSCE COUNSELLING CASE 9.4 – 'What is this ERCP thing you think I should have?'

Endoscopic retrograde cholangiopancreatography is a diagnostic and therapeutic procedure, usually performed by gastroenterologists or GI surgeons. A special side-viewing endoscope (duodenoscope) has channels through the instrument to allow cannulae and instruments to be guided into the biliary tree under direct vision or video monitoring. Radio-opaque dye can delineate the anatomy of the bile ducts, and identify common bile duct stones or strictures such as cancer. Electrocautery can enlarge the sphincter of Oddi ('sphincterotomy') and special baskets and crushing forceps can clear the duct of stones. Tumours can be biopsied by special forceps, or brushings of the duct for cytology can be obtained.

This procedure is a highly specialized area requiring dedicated equipment, and even with experts has a small failure rate. Complications are rare, but include bleeding or perforation (from sphincterotomy), pancreatitis (probably from high-pressure dye injection) and death in around 0.5 per cent.

APPENDICITIS

Q1: What is the likely differential diagnosis?
Q2: What issues in the given history support the diagnosis?
Q3: What additional features in the history would you seek to support a particular diagnosis?
Q4: What clinical examination would you perform and why?
Q5: What investigations would be most helpful and why?
Q6: What treatment options are appropriate?

Clinical cases

● CASE 9.7 – 'I've got a really bad pain in my right side.'

A 17-year-old man comes into A&E with a 12-hour history of nausea, lack of appetite and vague pain that is now becoming more severe and localized to the right side.

● CASE 9.8 – 'I've developed another episode of pain on the right.'

Moderate right-sided lower abdominal pain has brought a 24-year-old woman to the surgical assessment unit. She has had this on two previous occasions, with no diagnosis being made. The pain is constant, and makes her nauseated.

● CASE 9.9 – 'The pain is getting worse, and I've started to vomit.'

This 45-year-old businessman has delayed coming into hospital ('can't stand the place') and is now doubled over with severe pain, vomiting and rigors. When seen, he is tachycardic and has a palpable abdominal mass in the right iliac fossa.

ⁱⁱ OSCE Counselling Cases

OSCE COUNSELLING CASE 9.5 – 'I'm going to overwinter in the Antarctic. Should I have my appendix removed beforehand?'

A 32-year-old male meteorologist is planning to spend 6 months at a research station in the Antarctic; this sometimes becomes inaccessible to medical evacuation flights for up to a month at a time. He has heard that sometimes prophylactic appendicectomy is performed in this situation.

Q1: What would you advise?

OSCE COUNSELLING CASE 9.6 – 'Why has my wife developed complications after her appendicectomy?'

After having her appendix removed last week, a 44-year-old woman has started to feel progressively more unwell, with lower abdominal pain and fevers and diarrhoea. Her GP sends her back into hospital, where a pelvic abscess is diagnosed on abdominal CT.

Q1: What will you tell this woman about why this has happened?

 Key concepts

In order to work through the core clinical cases in this section, you will need to understand the following key concepts.

What is appendicitis?

Inflammation of the appendix is usually caused by obstruction of the lumen by a faecolith (a small hard ball of faecal material), with subsequent stasis, bacterial growth, impairment of the blood supply, necrosis of the wall and finally perforation if not treated promptly.

What happens if the appendix perforates?

The omentum has been described as the 'policeman of the gut', and tends to wall off serosal inflammation of the appendix. Perforation may be contained by the omentum (or other surrounding structures) to form a localized abscess. If this does not happen, generalized peritonitis is likely.

Answers

 CASE 9.7 – 'I've got a really bad pain in my right side.'

 Q1: What is the likely differential diagnosis?

A1

- Acute appendicitis

- Gastroenteritis

- Mesenteric adenitis

- Crohn's disease of the terminal ileum.

 Q2: What issues in the given history support the diagnosis?

A2

Appendicitis is typically preceded by a vague abdominal pain, because visceral inflammation is often poorly localized to the midline; organs derived from the midgut (like the appendix) usually have pain referred to the periumbilical region. As continued inflammation spreads to the serosal surface, and involves the body wall, the pain tends to localize to where the appendix is located. Nausea and anorexia go hand in hand with GI inflammation.

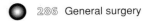 **Q3: What additional features in the history would you seek to support a particular diagnosis?**

A3

Has the patient had this type of pain previously? Recurrent pains are atypical of appendicitis ('grumbling' appendicitis, while beloved of GPs, probably does not exist). Check about other GI symptoms, particularly diarrhoea; in appendicitis, these usually follow the initial pain or discomfort.

Q4: What clinical examination would you perform and why?

A4

Abdominal examination should seek to differentiate tenderness (mild-to-moderate pain on palpation) from guarding (increased muscular tone) or peritonism (guarding with moderate-to-severe pain). Cough and percussion tenderness are hallmarks of peritonism, and with the appropriate history are often diagnostic of acute appendicitis. Rebound tenderness is unreliable and cruel, and should never be performed.

Digital rectal examination has been considered mandatory in suspected appendicitis in the past, but realistically adds little in most patients without a specific indication.

Repeated clinical examination is useful in borderline cases. A 12-hour period of observation with repeated examination is almost always safe, and better than operating in the middle of the night.

Q5: What investigations would be most helpful and why?

A5

- WCC and inflammatory markers (erythrocyte sedimentation rate [ESR], C-reactive protein [CRP]) are usually moderately raised in appendicitis. Other blood tests are normal.

- UTI can be excluded by midstream urine (MSU).

- Plain abdominal radiographs add little diagnostically. Limited CT of the right iliac fossa is highly sensitive and specific for appendicitis, but is usually not available.

 Q6: What treatment options are appropriate?

A6

- Supportive: no role.

- Medical: it is probable that broad-spectrum antibiotics alter the course of early appendicitis but, once serosal inflammation or ischaemia/necrosis of the wall has occurred, the appendix will progress to perforation unless removed. Antibiotics (one regimen is cefuroxime plus metronidazole) may be used prophylactically at operation to reduce wound infection, or as postoperative treatment if perforation has occurred.

- Surgical: appendicectomy is indicated. This is usually performed with an open incision in the right iliac fossa, although laparoscopic techniques are also used (particularly following a diagnostic laparoscopy; see next section).

 CASE 9.8 – 'I've developed another episode of pain on the right.'

 Q1: What is the likely differential diagnosis?

A1

- Non-specific abdominal pain

- Appendicitis

- Right-sided gynaecological pathology (ovarian cyst, pelvic inflammatory disease, ectopic pregnancy)

- Crohn's disease, gastroenteritis, biliary colic or cholecystitis (if gallbladder low).

Q2: What issues in the given history support the diagnosis?

A2

The previous episodes of pain suggest a recurring problem, although it is not unheard of to have similar episodes before frank acute appendicitis.

Q3: **What additional features in the history would you seek to support a particular diagnosis?**

A3

Could she be pregnant? A careful gynaecological and sexual history is mandatory in this situation. Urinary symptoms should also be elicited.

 Q4: **What clinical examination would you perform and why?**

A4

As well as abdominal examination, vaginal and pelvic examination should be performed. Masses, tenderness, vaginal discharge and cervical excitation should all be sought.

 Q5: **What investigations would be most helpful and why?**

A5

- Pregnancy test before almost anything else.

- Basic blood tests including WCC, haemoglobin (Hb), urea and electrolytes (U&Es).

- MSU to exclude UTI.

- Traditionally, ultrasonography (transvaginal being better than transabdominal) has been used for assessment of right iliac fossa pain in women. However, this frequently fails to lead to a diagnosis.

- Diagnostic laparoscopy is being used more aggressively in many units, e.g. if pain is not settling after overnight observation. It has the benefit of directly visualizing the pelvic organs and appendix, and the ability to proceed to a therapeutic procedure if appropriate.

 Q6: **What treatment options are appropriate?**

A6

- Supportive: fluids, analgesia and a period of 12 hours of observation are useful when the diagnosis is equivocal. Those with mild pain that resolves may then drink, eat, mobilize and be discharged without follow-up.

- Medical: no role, although antibiotics may be used when surgical delay is inevitable, e.g. in some rural communities.

- Surgical: operation is indicated for definite or deteriorating signs and symptoms. It is generally considered that a 'negative appendicectomy' (i.e. operating on and removing an uninflamed appendix) is a less dangerous option than prevaricating and allowing perforation, abscess or peritonitis.

CASE 9.9 – 'The pain is getting worse, and I've started to vomit.'

 Q1: What is the likely differential diagnosis?

A1

- Appendix mass
- Appendix abscess
- Perforated Crohn's disease or perforated caecal cancer.

 Q2: What issues in the given history support the diagnosis?

A2

This story is typical of 'missed' appendicitis; patients usually present within 24–48 hours of symptoms starting. If the appendix perforates, systemic signs of inflammation are often more severe.

 Q3: What additional features in the history would you seek to support a particular diagnosis?

A3

Gastrointestinal symptoms that have been present for a long period may point to underlying pathology such as inflammatory bowel disease (Crohn's disease). Neoplasms may be silent in the caecum as a result of liquid stool and large calibre of the bowel, but may result in iron-deficiency anaemia with consequent lethargy.

 Q4: What clinical examination would you perform and why?

A4

Abdominal examination has found a mass; confirm that it is tender, without hurting the patient. If it contains gas, it may be resonant to percussion.

 Q5: What investigations would be most helpful and why?

A5

Basic blood tests may show a markedly elevated WCC (only mildly raised in uncomplicated appendicitis). Anaemia may hint at a caecal neoplasm. Liver function tests (aspartate aminotransferase [AST]/alanine aminotransferase [ALT]) may be deranged if the patient is septic.

Plain abdominal films may show an ileus or frank bowel obstruction, and occasionally free gas is seen under the diaphragm on chest radiograph. Ultrasonography or CT of the abdomen is urgently indicated (i.e. same day), because it will determine emergency management.

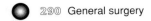

A6

- Supportive: fluid resuscitation and analgesia are needed.

- Medical: if an appendix mass (without abscess) is found, broad-spectrum antibiotics targeted against gut organisms should be given; ciprofloxacin and metronidazole is one suggested combination, usually given for 5 days. If the patient settles with this treatment, only 20 per cent develop 'recurrent' appendicitis. If an interval appendicectomy is not performed, any underlying bowel disease should be excluded with a colonoscopy or barium enema in those aged over 40 years old.

- Radiological: if a localized appendix abscess is present, percutaneous drainage with ultrasound or CT guidance may avoid an initial operation.

Surgery will be needed if the inflammation is localized (appendicectomy via the usual incision or midline laparotomy) or if generalized peritonitis is present (laparotomy to allow washout of the abdomen, with appendicectomy). Perforated Crohn's disease or cancer may require resection of a bowel segment – rejoining of the bowel may be unwise in the presence of severe infection, so a stoma may need to be brought to the body surface temporarily.

👥 OSCE Counselling Cases – Answers

OSCE COUNSELLING CASE 9.5 – 'I'm going to overwinter in the Antarctic. Should I have my appendix removed beforehand?'

A1

Appendicitis occurs in about 6 per cent of people over their lives, most often in the second or third decade. The risk in any 6-month period for an individual is quite small, and impossible to predict. One might naturally be concerned about such a possibility if access to medical care might be difficult. The risk of complications for an (potentially unnecessary) operation needs to be balanced against the risk of the illness itself very carefully.

Laparoscopic appendicectomy has probably reduced the morbidity of such procedures even further, and many surgeons would at least consider such a request in the appropriate circumstances.

OSCE COUNSELLING CASE 9.6 – 'Why has my wife developed complications after her appendicectomy?'

Medical interventions (and many investigative procedures) have the potential to cause harm as well as good. Informed consent should include information about common adverse events, as well as rare complications that may have a significant impact. Patients should always have ample opportunity to ask as much about their care as they feel appropriate. This is sometimes harder to do in the emergency situation.

Pelvic abscess is an uncommon but recognized complication of appendicitis. Appropriate medical care, including drainage and antibiotics, should minimize the risk of long-term sequelae.

COLON AND RECTAL CANCER

? Questions for each of the clinical case scenarios given

Q1: What is the likely differential diagnosis?
Q2: What issues in the given history support the diagnosis?
Q3: What additional features in the history would you seek to support a particular diagnosis?
Q4: What clinical examination would you perform and why?
Q5: What investigations would be most helpful and why?
Q6: What treatment options are appropriate?

Clinical cases

● CASE 9.10 – 'I've developed rectal bleeding.'

A 45-year-old woman has intermittently noticed some dark liquid blood and occasional blood clots in her bowel motions over the last 3 months. She is well otherwise and her bowel habit has not altered.

● CASE 9.11 – 'My bowel habit has changed.'

The 48-year-old husband of the same woman mentions that he is troubled by not passing a motion as frequently as usual, and when he does sometimes it seems looser. He once noticed some bright red blood on the toilet paper. He is worried because his older brother developed bowel cancer when he was in his late 40s.

● CASE 9.12 – 'It feels like I can't finish my bowel motion.'

A 74-year-old man has been complaining of intermittent colicky abdominal pains, with frequent dark blood in the stools. Over the last 2 months he has noticed that he feels 'funny' deep inside his pelvis when he passes a motion, and never feels like he has emptied properly. His trousers seem looser and he has had to punch another hole in his belt.

ȦȦ OSCE Counselling Cases

OSCE COUNSELLING CASE 9.7 – 'What do I need to know about colonoscopy?'

The 45-year-old woman in Case 9.10 had a colonoscopy organized, and was anxious about the procedure. She understood the need for the test, but heard that it was very painful.

Q1: What are the risks of colonoscopy?

OSCE COUNSELLING CASE 9.8 – 'Why are they talking about radiotherapy before my bowel cancer operation?'

A 66-year-old man with rectal bleeding and tenesmus is found to have a large, fixed mass on rectal examination. Biopsies confirm rectal cancer and MRI shows probable metastatic nodes in the mesorectum. A referral for preoperative radiotherapy is made.

Q1: What does radiotherapy add?

Q2: Are there any side effects that the patient needs to know about?

Key concepts

In order to work through the core clinical cases in this section, you will need to understand the following key concepts.

What is the difference between colon and rectal cancer?

Although these are technically the same disease – epithelial neoplasia of the lining of the large bowel – they present with a different spectrum of disease as a result of characteristics of the site. In the right colon, huge growth can occur with little in the way of symptoms, and anaemia is common. In the left colon, dark but noticeable bleeding may be the most common symptom. Rectal cancers occurring near the anus in the confined pelvis may have brighter bleeding or defecation symptoms (e.g. tenesmus, a feeling of incomplete evacuation).

Surgery and other treatments may differ markedly by site; radiotherapy is often used in the pelvis for rectal cancer, whereas chemotherapy may be used for advanced colon cancer.

What causes colon cancer?

There is now a well-defined pathway from normal colonic epithelium, to dysplastic changes in the cells, to early neoplasia (such as benign polyps) and subsequently to true malignancy – this is the so-called adenoma–carcinoma sequence. This pathway suggests that finding and treating benign polyps early may reduce the risk of later cancer. How might we do this?

What are the principles of treatment of colorectal cancer?

The aim of treatment should obviously be curative, but, where this is not possible, local control of disease is important. Obstruction and bleeding are the most important local complications of colorectal cancer and resection of the affected bowel (even in the presence of metastases) is usually appropriate. Chemotherapy and radiotherapy are important treatment modalities in specific situations; multidisciplinary assessment should be the rule rather than the exception.

Answers

CASE 9.10 – 'I've developed rectal bleeding.'

Q1: What is the likely differential diagnosis?

A1

- Haemorrhoids
- Proctitis/colitis
- Bleeding from polyp or cancer.

Q2: What issues in the given history support the diagnosis?

A2

With a non-specific history of bleeding that is not 'typically' haemorrhoidal (e.g. bright red, painless, only associated with defecation) in a patient aged over 40 years, other sources for the bleeding need to be considered and excluded. The lack of other symptoms makes serious pathology less likely, but remember that early cancer may have minimal symptoms.

Q3: What additional features in the history would you seek to support a particular diagnosis?

A3

Check for an alteration of bowel habit. Is there a family history of bowel cancer? If sinister causes for the bleeding are ultimately excluded, a careful dietary history may reveal too little fibre in the diet – this is a common theme in minor anorectal conditions.

Q4: What clinical examination would you perform and why?

A4

The critical examination is of the abdomen including a DRE. The subtleties of abdominal examination are not needed, but masses should be sought and identified. Initially proctoscopy and sigmoidoscopy may be omitted if equipment is suboptimal, but it is indefensible not to perform a rectal examination when rectal bleeding is the presenting complaint.

Q5: What investigations would be most helpful and why?

A5

If the index of suspicion for malignancy is low, rigid sigmoidoscopic examination (which actually best examines the rectum, not the sigmoid – in the USA, this is called a proctoscope [*procto* = rectum] and the UK proctoscope is called an anoscope;

this terminology is more accurate, but tradition rules), coupled with a barium enema to examine the remaining colon, may be adequate. A better investigation is colonoscopy, which examines the whole colon in about 90 per cent of patients, or flexible sigmoidoscopy, which views only the left colon. Both have therapeutic ability, in contrast to a barium enema. CT colonography may be more commonly used in the future.

Colonoscopy was performed in this woman, and showed four small polyps scattered through the colon, and one 2 cm pedunculated lesion in the distal left colon.

 Q6: What treatment options are appropriate?

A6

With the therapeutic ability of colonoscopy, the polyp was removed with a diathermy snare cauterizing through the stalk. The polyp was retrieved and sent for histology and showed a dysplastic polyp with no evidence of malignancy.

If the lesion had proven to be malignant, further treatment options would include advanced colonoscopic resection (uncommon) or surgical resection of the involved colon. Being benign, one should consider the need for further colonoscopy in the future – development of polyps makes further polyps more likely in future.

● CASE 9.11 – 'My bowel habit has changed.'

 Q1: What is the likely differential diagnosis?

A1

- Diverticular disease (diverticulosis)
- Colitis
- Left-sided colon cancer.

 Q2: What issues in the given history support the diagnosis?

A2

Alteration of bowel habit is always significant over the age of 40 years, but benign causes such as diverticulosis are more common than malignancy. Bleeding has not been a major feature, nor has pain or tenesmus (a feeling of incomplete evacuation). The family history of colorectal cancer is of note, although the increase in cancer risk from baseline is only moderate (three to six times).

 Q3: What additional features in the history would you seek to support a particular diagnosis?

A3

Some extracolonic cancers in family members may raise the possibility of hereditary non-polyposis colorectal cancer (HNPCC), including endometrial, ovarian, stomach and pancreas, so take a careful family history. Ask about weight change.

Q4: What clinical examination would you perform and why?

A4

Abdominal examination and DRE should be performed, followed by proctoscopy and sigmoidoscopy.

 Q5: What investigations would be most helpful and why?

A5

Colonoscopy is the best investigation in this situation, although double-contrast barium enema may be performed in some settings. Abdominal CT and CT colonography ('virtual' colonoscopy) are becoming more commonly used. Biopsy can be performed with colonoscopy if suspicious masses or polyps are encountered.

Barium enema was performed in this man as a result of resource limitations at his health-care facility. This showed severe diverticulosis in the sigmoid colon, with a comment that 'small polyps in the sigmoid colon could not be excluded as a result of the limitations of the study'. A subsequent flexible sigmoidoscopy of this area was performed and was normal.

 Q6: What treatment options are appropriate?

A6

- Supportive: given that there has been no complications of the diverticulosis, dietary management (with a high-fibre diet) may reduce the risk of progression of this acquired condition. Many patients will, however, ultimately progress and require specific treatment.

- Medical: antibiotics may be required for infective complications of diverticular disease, either diverticulitis or peri-diverticular abscess formation. (The latter may also be treated by percutaneous drainage under ultrasonic or CT guidance.) Free perforation with peritonitis usually requires emergency operation.

- Surgical: resection of the affected bowel segment (sigmoid colectomy) may be required in some patients, usually those with repeated hospitalizations or complications. Severe diverticulitis with perforation may require emergency surgery, either with a Hartmann procedure (resection of the diseased area with an end-colostomy; this may be joined up 6–12 months later) or resection and primary anastomosis after on-table colonic lavage.

● CASE 9.12 – 'It feels like I can't finish my bowel motion.'

Q1: What is the likely differential diagnosis?

A1

- Rectal cancer
- Left-sided colon cancer
- Severe diverticular disease.

Q2: What issues in the given history support the diagnosis?

A2

This history sounds ominous: the 'funny' feeling is called tenesmus and is characteristic of advanced rectal cancer. Weight loss with objective findings as described is an important symptom.

 Q3: What additional features in the history would you seek to support a particular diagnosis?

A3

Again, a family history should be obtained. A thorough history (and particularly systems enquiry) will be required as a major operation may be needed.

 Q4: What clinical examination would you perform and why?

A4

Abdominal and rectal examination, with proctoscopy and sigmoidoscopy, should be performed. This reveals a large hard rectal mass, and the liver is palpable and craggy. General examination is required to detect any other significant findings.

 Q5: What investigations would be most helpful and why?

A5

A number of investigations are necessary. Biopsy of the mass may be done in the clinic, but is often done as part of an examination under anaesthetic to determine tumour situation and fastness to surrounding structures. CT of the pelvis and abdomen and MRI of the pelvis are often performed, with some centres also using endorectal ultrasonography or other specialized imaging techniques. Colonoscopy should be performed to check for other polyps or tumours (synchronous lesions).

 Q6: What treatment options are appropriate?

A6

- Supportive: nutrition is important and should be optimized. In widespread disease, or when curative treatment is declined by the patient, palliative care measures such as pain relief are of critical importance.

- Medical: little role.

- Surgical: treatment is attempted with curative or palliative intent. Resection of the tumour is performed either through the abdomen (anterior resection [of the rectum], sometimes with a temporary protective ileostomy), or via a combined approach taking out the tumour and the anal canal in the perineum to leave a permanent end-colostomy (abdominoperineal resection [of the rectum]). This may be done even in the presence of liver metastases in order to minimize symptoms in the future. Rarely, resection of colorectal metastases in the liver is performed.

● Other: radiotherapy to the tumour in the pelvis may be performed as an extra (adjuvant) treatment combined with surgery, and may be done before the operation to shrink the tumour or to reduce the incidence of local recurrence. If the tumour cannot be removed, or the patient declines surgery, primary treatment with radiotherapy may provide palliative benefit. Chemotherapy has a limited role in rectal cancer.

♛♛ OSCE Counselling Cases – Answers

OSCE COUNSELLING CASE 9.7 – 'What do I need to know about colonoscopy?'

A1

Colonoscopy is usually a safe procedure, but a number of issues need to be discussed. These include risks related to the procedure itself and those related to the sedation that usually accompanies colonoscopy.

Perforation is extremely rare with diagnostic colonoscopy, and rises (but is still uncommon) with interventional procedures such as polypectomy. Perforation is usually treated with antibiotics and active observation; surgery is rarely needed and death from colonoscopy is almost unheard of. Significant bleeding is again very rare.

Failure of the procedure to obtain the information should be discussed. Rates of complete examination (sometimes including intubation of the ileocaecal valve to visualize the terminal ileum) vary with experience but exceed 95 per cent in many places. Despite excellent technique, lesions may sometimes be missed.

Operative risks specific to this procedure may be early or late.

Specific risks to consider in groin hernia repair are recurrence of hernia (i.e. failure of treatment), scrotal haematoma, impairment of vascular supply to testicle (ischaemic orchitis) and late neuralgic pain from the wound.

Patients usually need to make a choice about whether to proceed with an operation based on their assessment of the risks of the procedure versus the risks of the underlying condition. The best source of this information is the medical team, based on published evidence (where present) or best opinions. There is a strong consensus that groin hernia should usually be repaired surgically when present.

OSCE COUNSELLING CASE 9.8 – 'Why are they talking about radiotherapy before my bowel cancer operation?'

A1

Preoperative radiotherapy is used either where tumour shrinkage ('down-staging') is required to convert a borderline resectable tumour to one that can confidently be removed, or to minimize the chance of local recurrence in operable but advanced disease (i.e. invasion through the rectal wall or nodal involvement on imaging). A number of studies have now shown a major reduction in local recurrence when preoperative radiotherapy is used appropriately.

A2

Radiotherapy risks can be considered as general and site specific. Common general side effects include tiredness (the reason for which is poorly understood) and a local skin reaction such as sunburn.

Site-specific radiotherapy issues in the pelvis may include vaginal dryness in women, and impotence in men. The latter may respond to agents such as sildenafil (Viagra). Most radiotherapy avoids the gonads and should not impair fertility. However, sperm banking is an option for some to consider. Bladder or bowel inflammation can occur with radiotherapy, and some degree of the latter is inevitable. In extreme cases, a diverting colostomy may be considered.

Late side effects can also occur and should be carefully discussed by the radiation oncologist.

SURGICAL EMERGENCIES

? Questions for each of the clinical case scenarios given

Q1: What is the likely differential diagnosis?
Q2: What issues in the given history support the diagnosis?
Q3: What additional features in the history would you seek to support a particular diagnosis?
Q4: What clinical examination would you perform and why?
Q5: What investigations would be most helpful and why?
Q6: What treatment options are appropriate?

Clinical cases

CASE 9.13 – An acute abdomen.

A 70-year-old man is brought into A&E complaining of abdominal pain. Over the last few months he had noted a change in bowel habit and a loss of weight. On examination he is pale, tachycardic and hypotensive, and his abdomen is rigid on palpation.

CASE 9.14 – Bowel obstruction.

A 60-year-old woman presents with a 2-day history of abdominal distension, pain, profuse bilious vomiting and constipation.

Answers

 CASE 9.13 – An acute abdomen.

 Q1: What is the likely differential diagnosis?

A1

This man has an acute abdomen. The most likely diagnosis is a perforated viscus (probably colon). Other common causes include pancreatitis, ruptured abdominal aneurysm, ischaemic bowel and non-surgical causes (myocardial infarct, lower lobe pneumonia and diabetic ketoacidosis).

 Q2: What issues in the given history support the diagnosis?

A2

The age of this man and a history of a change in bowel habit plus weight loss suggest a left-sided colonic neoplasm. The sudden onset of pain could indicate a perforation, probably at the site of the tumour. If the tumour has been causing an obstruction, the perforation can occur at a more proximal part of the colon – typically the caecum (the thinnest and widest part of the large bowel and therefore the most easily distended). This requires a patent ileocaecal valve – producing a closed loop obstruction. Right iliac fossa pain may be a warning of impending perforation in such cases and requires action. Severe diverticular disease can cause a colonic perforation but does not usually cause weight loss. Free gas on the plain radiographs and an acute abdomen will also be seen with a perforated duodenal ulcer, but is normally accompanied by a history of peptic ulcer disease and patients tend to be less septic than those with a faecal peritonitis.

 Q3: What additional features in the history would you seek to support a particular diagnosis?

A3

Other factors that would point towards a colonic cancer include: any passage of fresh blood mixed in with the stool, a family history of bowel and related cancers, previous colon cancer or inflammatory bowel disease.

Q4: What clinical examination would you perform and why?

A4

A full examination should be undertaken. Abdominal examination would be performed to assess which area is most tender. Digital rectal examination may reveal a rectal tumour and should always be performed. A rigid, quiet abdomen would suggest generalized peritonitis. A palpable node in the left supraclavicular area would suggest disseminated intra-abdominal neoplasia.

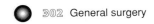

Q5: What investigations would be most helpful and why?

A5

An FBC may show anaemia secondary to bleeding from the tumour. Arterial blood gases would give an indication of the degree of metabolic acidosis. Clotting parameters may be abnormal in the severely septic patient. Amylase and glucose levels should be checked in all patients with an acute abdomen.

An erect chest radiograph may show free gas under the diaphragm, but its absence does not rule out a perforation. An abdominal plain film may also show free gas. An abdominal CT can be performed if the patient is stable and there is some confusion over the diagnosis.

Q6: What treatment options are appropriate?

A6

Initially the patient would be fluid resuscitated with several litres of colloid. Oxygen would be given via a facemask and a urinary catheter is inserted to aid fluid management. A wide-bore nasogastric tube should be inserted if the patient is vomiting. Thromboembolic deterrent stockings (TEDSs) should be applied. Opiate analgesia is given regularly. Low-molecular-weight heparin should be given because of the high risk of thrombosis, but should be discussed with the anaesthetist depending on the use of an epidural for postoperative pain management.

This patient requires surgery to treat the problem but all effort should be taken to optimize the patient, preferably in a high dependency unit. The safest surgical option for a sigmoid perforation would be Hartmann's procedure (sigmoid colectomy, closure of rectal stump and formation of an end-colostomy). An alternative to this would be a resection of the sigmoid, an on-table washout of the remaining colon and a primary anastomosis. This removes the need for a stoma and secondary reversal procedure but does risk anastomotic breakdown and leak.

Faecal peritonitis carries a high mortality rate and good communication with the patient and family should ensure that they are aware of this before surgery.

CASE 9.14 – Bowel obstruction.

Q1: What is the likely differential diagnosis?

A1

The most likely diagnosis is a bowel obstruction (probably small bowel). The common causes for this include adhesions, hernias, malignancy and volvulus.

Q2: What issues in the given history support the diagnosis?

A2

The classic symptoms of small bowel obstruction (SBO) are the four symptoms given. The presence of profuse, bilious and frequent vomiting suggests that this is caused by obstruction in the small bowel. If the vomiting were faeculent and intermittent, a large bowel obstruction should be suspected (this requires a non-functioning ileocaecal valve to allow back flow).

Q3: What additional features in the history would you seek to support a particular diagnosis?

A3

The history would be aiming to assess the site of the obstruction (e.g. the patient with proximal SBO tends to have very profuse, bilious vomiting and minimal distension, and can still be passing stool) and the cause. A history of previous abdominal surgery, especially for abdominal malignancy, could be relevant.

 Q4: What clinical examination would you perform and why?

A4

The examination may reveal the presence of an obstructing hernia. The degree of tenderness, especially localized, may indicate impending bowel perforation in a closed-loop obstruction. Bowel sounds may be 'tinkling' or absent.

 Q5: What investigations would be most helpful and why?

A5

A plain abdominal film will show dilated small bowel loops, occasionally with an obvious cut-off point. Arterial blood gases may show some metabolic acidosis if the bowel blood supply is compromised. These can be difficult to interpret as a result of the presence of a metabolic alkalosis secondary to vomiting. A contrast follow-through may be useful to differentiate between partial and complete obstruction.

 Q6: What treatment options are appropriate?

A6

Fluid resuscitation is essential because of the large volume of fluid lost into the bowel lumen (third space loss). A wide-bore nasogastric tube will decompress the bowel. In a patient with no history of abdominal surgery or if an obstructing hernia is identified, surgery should be performed after optimization. In those with suspected adhesional obstruction and no physiological or biochemical evidence of bowel ischaemia, a period of intravenous fluids and nasogastric drainage (drip and suck) can be undertaken to see whether it resolves spontaneously.

VASCULAR: AORTIC ANEURYSM

Q1: What is the likely differential diagnosis?
Q2: What issues in the given history support the diagnosis?
Q3: What additional features in the history would you seek to support a particular diagnosis?
Q4: What clinical examination would you perform and why?
Q5: What investigations would be most helpful and why?
Q6: What treatment options are appropriate?

Clinical cases

● CASE 9.15 – 'I thought I had gallstones. What is an aneurysm?'

A 55-year-old publican was sent by his GP for ultrasonography for suspected gallstones. The report shows no gallstones, but comment is made about a 4.5 cm abdominal aortic aneurysm.

● CASE 9.16 – 'My doctor tells me that I need an operation on my aneurysm.'

The same patient has regular repeat scans. Three years later, the aneurysm has grown to 6.0 cm. He is referred to a vascular surgeon; she recommends an operation to repair the aneurysm.

● CASE 9.17 – Severe back pain and collapse with a known aneurysm.

A patient in the same practice is also known to have an aneurysm, measuring 6.0 cm in diameter. He was reluctant to have an operation. He has had back pain for 2 days, which became severe this morning. Visiting the practice for pain relief, he suddenly becomes clammy, yells in pain and collapses. An ambulance is called.

👥 OSCE Counselling Cases

OSCE COUNSELLING CASE 9.9 – 'What about this "stenting" I've heard about?'

A 57-year-old woman with a 5.5 cm aortic aneurysm has had treatment recommended to her. She does an internet search and finds that there is a new treatment where the aneurysm is stented from the inside of the vessel, with almost immediate recovery. Can she have this treatment instead?

OSCE COUNSELLING CASE 9.10 – 'It's not that serious. I couldn't die from this operation, could I?'

As part of the counselling and consent process, a patient becomes very concerned that he might die from the operation. Surely this can't be common?

Key concepts

In order to work through the core clinical cases in this section, you will need to understand the following key concepts.

Definition

This is a permanent localized dilatation (> 1.5 times normal) of an artery. A true aneurysm involves all vessel wall layers (intima, media, adventitia), whereas a false aneurysm is a contained haematoma caused by disruption of the wall or leak from an anastomosis.

Risk factors for aortic aneurysm

Although most aneurysms are thought to be a reflection of atherosclerosis (with the usual risk factors of smoking, hypertension, diabetes, etc.), there is some evidence that it is a separate arterial disease. Elderly men who have brothers with an aneurysm have a high incidence. The presence of popliteal or femoral aneurysms is a warning flag; they often coexist.

What is the natural history?

The expansion rate of aneurysms is variable in individual patients, but most will enlarge with time at around 0.5 cm each year. Rupture is uncommon below 5.5 cm and the patient is generally observed. The risk of rupture increases disproportionately with increasing size.

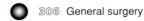
Answers

 CASE 9.15 – 'I thought I had gallstones. What is an aneurysm?'

 Q1: What is the likely differential diagnosis?

A1

Although the diagnosis is clear, the aetiology has a differential diagnosis. Most aneurysms are degenerative; atherosclerosis is usually present but not causative. Rarely pancreatitis or trauma can be a predisposing factor, as can syphilis (now historical), other infections (TB) and connective tissue disorders.

 Q2: What issues in the given history support the diagnosis?

A2

Male sex, age over 65, hypertension and smoking are the most important predisposing factors.

 Q3: What additional features in the history would you seek to support a particular diagnosis?

A3

Other manifestations of cardiovascular disease include coronary artery disease and peripheral vascular disease (PVD), both of which have classic symptoms. There is a high rate of aneurysms in siblings (especially brothers) and this should be asked about. Some suggest that any brothers be screened for the presence of aneurysms.

 Q4: What clinical examination would you perform and why?

A4

Full cardiovascular and peripheral vascular examination should be performed including a BP measurement. Clinical examination should include careful and gentle palpation of the abdomen – an aneurysm is characterized by 'expansile pulsation' (where the examining fingers of both hands move laterally apart as well as anteriorly in time with the pulse). Aneurysms may also occur in the same patient in the iliac, femoral and popliteal arteries, so these should also be checked.

Q5: What investigations would be most helpful and why?

A5

After detecting an aneurysm clinically or with ultrasonography, CT should be performed only if symptomatic or surgery is being considered. Ultrasonography can be used subsequently for monitoring. Investigations should be aimed at assessing predisposing factors. An ECG, cholesterol level, blood glucose and renal function should be assessed.

Q6: What treatment options are appropriate?

A6

For a small aneurysm (< 5.5 cm), observation is appropriate, with ultrasonography on a regular basis. Only 0.5 per cent will rupture in any particular year, so the risk of this watch-and-wait approach is generally smaller than the risk of an operation. Risk factor management is vital in such patients including controlling hypertension, hyperlipidaemia, diabetes and weight. Patients can be started on aspirin.

● CASE 9.16 – 'My doctor tells me I need an operation on my aneurysm.'

 Q1: What is the likely differential diagnosis?

 Q2: What issues in the given history support the diagnosis?

 Q3: What additional features in the history would you seek to support a particular diagnosis?

 Q4: What clinical examination would you perform and why?

A1–A4

As for Case 9.15.

 Q5: What investigations would be most helpful and why?

A5

Computed tomography should be performed to disclose the maximal size, the configuration of the aneurysm and, importantly, whether the origins of the renal arteries are involved (suprarenal aneurysm) or normal (infrarenal aneurysm). The former is less common but poses a much more complex problem. More extensive assessment of fitness for surgery should be undertaken to ensure that the patient is as fit as possible (e.g. cardiac stress test, respiratory function tests, cardiac echocardiography).

Q6: What treatment options are appropriate?

A6

- There is a 40 per cent chance of rupture over the next 5-year period, and the average survival without treatment is about 18 months. Options should be chosen with this in mind.

- Do nothing at patient choice, or if the anaesthetic and operative risks are thought to outweigh the benefits.

- Conventional operation: the aneurysmal segment of the aorta is replaced with a synthetic graft (Dacron) by laparotomy. Death from the operation occurs in 5–8 per cent of patients.

- Endoluminal stenting: a new technique suitable for some patients. Expanding stents are introduced via the femoral arteries and carefully positioned inside the aneurysm. This technique is rapidly evolving.

● CASE 9.17 – Severe back pain and collapse with a known aneurysm.

 Q1: What is the likely differential diagnosis?

A1

Rupture of the aneurysm is most likely and must be assumed.

Other intra-abdominal catastrophes may mimic ruptured aneurysm: perforated ulcer in someone with known abdominal aortic aneurysm (AAA); severe acute right heart failure with pulsatile tender hepatomegaly and pancreatitis.

 Q2: What issues in the given history support the diagnosis?

A2

The prodromal pain of a contained leak is not uncommon. In the face of a known aneurysm, acute severe abdominal pain demands immediate attention.

 Q3: What additional features in the history would you seek to support a particular diagnosis?

A3

It is unlikely that further history taking in this emergency situation would be helpful. A history from a family member may be useful to ensure that inappropriate surgery is not attempted (e.g. if the patient has an advanced incurable malignancy).

Q4: What clinical examination would you perform and why?

A4

Clinical examination in this setting may reveal a pulsatile abdominal mass, but the absence of such a finding should not dissuade emergency investigation and treatment. It is not uncommon for the abdomen to be rigid.

Q5: What investigations would be most helpful and why?

A5

Emergency CT may be considered if the patient is stable, but this should be only on the request of the operating vascular surgeon. All patients should have blood taken for cross-matching (10 units initially plus fresh frozen plasma [FFP]). In most centres, the patient would be taken to theatre for an emergency operation without any delays such as CT.

 Q6: What treatment options are appropriate?

A6

Initial management should **not** include aggressive fluid resuscitation because this leads to greater blood loss by displacing any clot present at the site of the rupture. A systolic pressure of 90–110 mmHg is optimum. The only effective treatment for a ruptured aortic aneurysm is emergency repair. Rupture is highly lethal: as a rule of thumb, about half of the patients die on the scene, half of the remainder die en route to hospital or in A&E, and half of those who make it to theatre subsequently die.

👥 OSCE Counselling Cases – Answers

OSCE COUNSELLING CASE 9.9 – 'What about this "stenting" I've heard about?'

Aortic stenting involves a vascular surgeon and/or radiologist inserting a balloon-inflated covered tube into the inside of the weakened and dilated aortic wall, usually via a small incision in the groin. Placement is assisted using radiological guidance. Although it can be faster and less invasive than open surgical treatment, stenting is not suitable for all patients as a result of the aneurysm morphology. As a relatively new form of treatment, long-term outcomes are not known. In addition, some new complications ('endo-leak') are recognized. There is a risk of on-table rupture during the procedure so patients must be warned that a conversion to open surgery may be required. Only a few centres offer this form of treatment, usually as part of a national trial.

OSCE COUNSELLING CASE 9.10 – 'It's not that serious. I couldn't die from this operation, could I?'

Depending on a number of factors, around 5–8 per cent of patients die from elective aortic aneurysm repair, and important complications may occur in around 20 per cent. Both morbidity and mortality numbers can be modified – excellent surgeons in excellent centres may achieve very good results, but selecting lower-risk patients will also appear to give the same outcome.

Any operative and anaesthetic risk should be weighed against the risk of the disease itself. A 6 cm aneurysm has about a 40 per cent risk of rupture (with its high attendant mortality) over 5 years, and the median survival of a group of patients with such an aneurysm is around 18 months.

PERIPHERAL VASCULAR DISEASE (PVD)

? Questions for each of the clinical case scenarios given

Q1: What is the likely differential diagnosis?
Q2: What issues in the given history support the diagnosis?
Q3: What additional features in the history would you seek to support a particular diagnosis?
Q4: What clinical examination would you perform and why?
Q5: What investigations would be most helpful and why?
Q6: What treatment options are appropriate?

Clinical cases

● CASE 9.18 – A 78-year-old man presents complaining of calf pain on walking.

A 78-year-old retired male teacher presents complaining of calf cramp in both legs on walking. This is worse on walking up an incline. The pain disappears after a short rest period. This has been occurring for the last 3 months and does not appear to be worsening.

● CASE 9.19 – The same man presents to A&E with an acutely painful leg.

Clinically his leg is pale and cold.

⚬━ Key concepts

In order to work through the core clinical cases in this section, you will need to understand the following key concepts.

Natural history

● Intermittent claudication affects 5 per cent of men over 50 years of age.

● 5 per cent of those with claudication progress to critical ischaemia in a year.

● 75 per cent of those with claudication remain stable or improve.

Critical leg ischaemia

● Persistently recurring ischaemic rest pain requiring regular adequate analgesia for > 2 weeks

● Ulceration or gangrene of the foot or toes, with an ankle pressure of < 50 mmHg or toe pressures of < 30 mmHg

Vascular imaging

Non-invasive imaging using duplex scanning (combining ultrasonography and Doppler images) and MR angiography (MRA) has expanded as a result of the quality of the information and safety.

Digital subtraction angiography (DSA) is performed by a catheter being inserted into the opposite femoral vessels to the limb being examined. This is then directed over the bifurcation to the other side (the Seldinger technique). The presence of a catheter has the benefit of allowing therapeutic procedures to be undertaken such as angioplasty or inserting a stent.

Answers

 CASE 9.18 – **A 78-year-old man presents complaining of calf pain on walking.**

 Q1: What is the likely differential diagnosis?

A1

- Peripheral vascular disease (PVD)
- Spinal stenosis.

 Q2: What issues in the given history support the diagnosis?

A2

The most likely cause will be PVD caused by atherosclerosis to the vessels to the lower limbs. The site of the stenosis or occlusion will affect the presenting symptoms. The proximal disease (e.g. common iliac) may produce buttock claudication on exercise as well as lower limb pain. The most common site to be affected is the obturator foramen (two-thirds of the way down the thigh). This produces classic intermittent claudication (IC). The important aspects to obtain are the distance walked before having to stop (remember that most patients and doctors are poor at judging this), the time required for the pain to resolve and walking to recommence, and an assessment of the nature of the problem (static or progressive).

Spinal stenosis causes a similar presentation, making differentiation between the two sometimes tricky. Lower limb pain from spinal stenosis tends to occur after varying distances walked and does not resolve within a few minutes of rest (unlike in IC). The subsequent distances may become shorter and the time for resolution of the pain increases. The patient may also complain of a 'bad' back with neurological symptoms.

 Q3: What additional features in the history would you seek to support a particular diagnosis?

A3

The diagnosis may be supported by the fact that the individual has risk factors that predispose him to atherosclerosis and he may also have other cardiovascular problems.

 Q4: What clinical examination would you perform and why?

A4

Full cardiovascular and peripheral vascular examination should be performed. The lower limbs may show signs of muscle wasting, thinning of the skin, loss of hair and ulceration. Peripheral pulses may be felt at the groin but are absent distally.

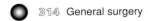 **Q5: What investigations would be most helpful and why?**

A5

In an individual not showing any signs of critical ischaemia or disabling claudication the investigations undertaken would be aimed at preventing disease progression and not treating the stenosis or occlusion. Ankle brachial pressure indices (ABPIs) should be recorded to allow quantitative comparison at future follow-up.

 Q6: What treatment options are appropriate?

A6

Cardiac function should be optimized to decrease any 'pump failure' as a cause. Strategies to slow disease progression should be undertaken (cessation of smoking, controlling hyperlipidaemia, good diabetic control). Anti-platelet medication should be started to prevent thrombosis of the vessel.

Regular exercise improves neovascularization and cardiorespiratory function, and helps weight loss.

 CASE 9.19 – The same man presents to A&E with an acutely painful leg.

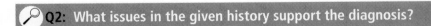 **Q1: What is the likely differential diagnosis?**

A1

The patient appears to have developed acute limb ischaemia (ALI). This is commonly the result of either thrombosis of diseased vessels or an embolus occluding the vessel. In a known sufferer of PVD the most likely cause is thrombosis.

Q2: What issues in the given history support the diagnosis?

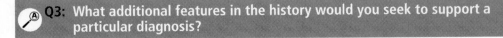 **Q3: What additional features in the history would you seek to support a particular diagnosis?**

A2, A3

Emboli need a source (the most common being thrombus within a fibrillating left atrium). Another clue to an embolus as a cause is the presence of normal pulses on the contralateral limb. The known presence of a popliteal aneurysm would point towards a thrombosis if now impalpable.

Q4: What clinical examination would you perform and why?

A4

An examination will need to assess the viability of the limb and the urgency for any intervention. Sensory and motor function should be assessed and recorded. ABPIs should be performed. The patient's general state should be assessed because ALI is often a pre-morbid episode and surgical intervention may cause unnecessary suffering.

The viability of the peripheral veins should be noted because these are typically used in bypass grafts.

 Q5: What investigations would be most helpful and why?

A5

Imaging of the arterial anatomy is required to identify the site and length of occlusion and the presence of distal vessels (suitable for a graft to be attached).

 Q6: What treatment options are appropriate?

A6

Depending on suitability, a bypass graft may be attempted to restore flow. If the limb is unsalvageable then an amputation may be required.

VASCULAR: CAROTID

? Questions for the clinical case scenario given

Q1: What is the likely differential diagnosis?
Q2: What issues in the given history support the diagnosis?
Q3: What additional features in the history would you seek to support a particular diagnosis?
Q4: What clinical examination would you perform and why?
Q5: What investigations would be most helpful and why?
Q6: What treatment options are appropriate?

Clinical case

CASE 9.20 – A previously well 39-year-old man attends A&E with a left-sided headache and slight word-finding difficulty after a mild whiplash injury 2 hours earlier.

He says the right arm doesn't 'feel right'. His wife has noticed a slight drooping of the eyelid on the left.

Answer

 CASE 9.20 – **A previously well 39-year-old man attends A&E with a left-sided headache and slight word-finding difficulty after a mild whiplash injury 2 hours earlier.**

 Q1: **What is the likely differential diagnosis?**

A1

- Dissection of the left carotid artery
- Left-sided intracerebral haemorrhage
- Migraine with aura
- Cerebrovascular disease causing a left-sided stroke in the middle cerebral artery territory
- The most likely cause is a dissection of the left carotid artery.

 Q2: **What issues in the given history support the diagnosis?**

A2

Carotid artery dissection is a significant cause of stroke in patients younger than 40 years. Dissections are usually subadventitial (between the media and adventitia or within the media), creating a false lumen that can cause stenosis, occlusion or pseudoaneurysm of the vessel. Simultaneously, the dissection may cause the formation of a thrombus from which fragments embolize. Strokes resulting from carotid dissection thus may have a haemodynamic or embolic origin.

As in this case, carotid artery dissections have non-specific presenting symptoms such as neurological deficits and headache. They often occur at a relatively young age and in previously healthy individuals, either spontaneously or after various degrees of trauma.

In this case a major clue to the cause of this patient's stroke is that he has a painful drooping left eyelid that suggests the possibility of Horner's syndrome. Horner's syndrome is caused by damage to the sympathetic supply to the eye. The sympathetic fibres travel with the carotid artery and carotid dissection may damage these fibres. A Horner's syndrome consists of ptosis, miosis, enophthalmos and sometimes loss of sweating on one half of the face. It is important to consider a carotid dissection in any case of painful Horner's syndrome.

The patient is very young to have significant cerebrovascular disease. The other causes mentioned would not generally be expected to cause Horner's syndrome, but remain possibilities.

 Q3: **What additional features in the history would you seek to support a particular diagnosis?**

A3

If the patient does not have a previous or family history of migraine this reduces the possibility of migrainous aetiology.

Q4: **What clinical examination would you perform and why?**

A4

Signs of an upper motoneuron pattern sensory–motor deficit in the right arm and signs of a Horner's syndrome (see above) should be found. It is also important to search for evidence of a head injury and, given the history of neck pain, to exclude evidence of spinal cord damage (bilateral limb weakness and sensory loss).

 Q5: **What investigations would be most helpful and why?**

A5

- CT/MRI of brain
- Non-invasive angiography of the carotid arteries
- Invasive contrast arteriography.

Computed tomography of the brain will be adequate in most circumstances to demonstrate ischaemic damage in the middle cerebral artery distribution, although MRI is more sensitive. Ultrasonography of carotid arteries is fast, convenient, non-invasive and highly sensitive, and may identify a dissection. Invasive contrast arteriography is more accurate but carries greater risk. Non-invasive alternatives include CT and MRA. ECG and echocardiography may be performed to rule out a cardiac source of the emboli.

 Q6: **What treatment options are appropriate?**

A6

- Aspirin
- Anticoagulation.

Formal anticoagulation for a period of months is often used, although the evidence base for this is relatively poor. In practice the choice between anticoagulation agents and aspirin is made, dependent on various circumstances (e.g. how severe the stroke is, the length of time since the dissection).

VENOUS DISEASE

? Questions for the clinical case scenario given

Q1: What is the likely differential diagnosis?
Q2: What issues in the given history support the diagnosis?
Q3: What additional features in the history would you seek to support a particular diagnosis?
Q4: What clinical examination would you perform and why?
Q5: What investigations would be most helpful and why?
Q6: What treatment options are appropriate?

Clinical case

○ **CASE 9.21 – A 65-year-old woman has noticed a breakdown in the skin over her left lower leg.**

The lower limb is swollen and discoloured.

🔑 Key concepts

In order to work through the core clinical cases in this section, you will need to understand the following key concepts.

What is an ulcer?

It is a lesion on the surface of the skin or a mucous surface resulting in epi-/endothelial loss produced by the sloughing of inflammatory necrotic tissue

What causes a venous ulcer?

● Venous disease

● Arterial disease

● Neuropathy, e.g. secondary to diabetes

● Malignancy

● Underlying osteomyelitis

● Inflammatory, e.g. pyoderma gangrenosum

● Vasculitis.

Venous ulceration is a result of an increase in the venous pressure of the lower limb. Over time this leads to changes seen to the 'gaiter' region of the leg. Chronic venous insufficiency is a term used to describe these changes, which are characterized by pigmentation, lipodermatosclerosis (thickening of the skin), swelling, varicose eczema and ulceration. The cause of this increased pressure is abnormalities to the flow caused by incompetent veins within this venous system, which can result from a previous deep vein thrombosis (DVT).

Answers

 CASE 9.21 – **A 65-year-old woman has noticed a breakdown in the skin over her left lower leg.**

 Q1: What is the likely differential diagnosis?

 Q2: What issues in the given history support the diagnosis?

A1, A2

Ulceration over the lower limb is a common problem with venous ulceration accounting for about 1 per cent of the NHS budget

With unilateral discoloration and swelling, the most likely cause is chronic venous insufficiency. A mixed arteriovenous condition should also be considered. Symptoms are exacerbated in elderly people by poor mobility, poor calf muscle pump and dependency.

Consider trauma and cellulitis.

Q3: What additional features in the history would you seek to support a particular diagnosis?

A3

The patient commonly remembers a trivial injury to the area that seemed to precipitate the ulcer. There may be a long history of varicose veins, possibly with previous surgery and a family history of varicose veins. The history may demonstrate either a known or risk factors predisposing to a DVT (e.g. lower limb immobilization within a plaster of Paris). Other factors that may affect wound healing such as poor nutritional state, renal impairment, use of steroids and diabetes are not uncommon in elderly people.

Q4: What clinical examination would you perform and why?

A4

A full venous examination must be performed with the patient standing. Abdominal examination should exclude pelvic/abdominal mass.

Emphasize the peripheral pulses.

Q5: What investigations would be most helpful and why?

A5

- A non-invasive assessment of the venous system of the limb should be performed. This will assess deep vein patency and competence as well as saphenofemoral, saphenopopliteal and perforator competence. This assessment is most commonly by duplex; however, hand-held Doppler in the outpatient clinic may be of use.

- ABPI assessment is required if there is any suggestion of arterial disease (because it may require compression). Arteriography may be required if arterial disease present.

- If an atypical ulcer consider biopsy (vasculitic ulcer, Marjolin's ulcer).

- Assessment of oedema.

 Q6: What treatment options are appropriate?

A6

Initial treatment will involve compression of the lower limb with four-layer compression bandages. Leg elevation is recommended when sitting or lying. Surgery should be considered in those with a patent deep venous system, but incompetence of the saphenofemoral, sphenopopliteal and/or perforators. Surgery does not increase speed of ulcer healing but reduces recurrence rates.

Nutritional and vitamin supplementation may be required as well as optimization of any medical problems. Patient education is essential to reduce recurrence.

BREAST

? Questions for each of the clinical case scenarios given

Q1: What is the likely differential diagnosis?
Q2: What issues in the given history support the diagnosis?
Q3: What additional features in the history would you seek to support a particular diagnosis?
Q4: What clinical examination would you perform and why?
Q5: What investigations would be most helpful and why?
Q6: What treatment options are appropriate?

Clinical Cases

● CASE 9.21 – 'I've found a breast lump.'

You are asked to see a 24 year old legal assistant who has noticed a lump in her breast over the last six weeks. She has not previously had breast lumps, and there is no family history of breast cancer. Examination reveals a 2 cm diameter firm mass lateral to her left nipple.

● CASE 9.22 – 'Something has shown up on my screening mammogram.'

A 53 year old woman is recalled for further imaging after her screening mammogram shows some 'calcifications'. A physical examination is unremarkable, with no lump palpable. A mammographic-guided stereotactic core biopsy is obtained, and histology shows ductal carcinoma *in situ* (DCIS). Appropriate treatment needs to be arranged.

● CASE 9.23 – 'I've found a lump under my armpit.'

When this 62 year old woman discovers a hard lump under her right arm, she sees her GP the next day, and is referred to a specialist Breast Unit. The finding is confirmed, and a hard 4 cm mass is also found deep to the nipple—the clinical impression is of breast cancer. Fine-needle aspiration cytology confirms malignant cells, and mammographic and ultrasound appearances support the diagnosis. Treatment options are discussed.

👥 OSCE Counselling Cases

OSCE COUNSELLING CASE 9.11 – 'What can I do for this breast pain?'

OSCE COUNSELLING CASE 9.12 – 'I'm confused by my surgical options for breast cancer. Which should I choose?'

🔑 Key concepts

In order to work through the core clinical cases in this chapter, you will need to understand the following key concepts:

How common is breast cancer?

Breast cancer is one of the most common female malignancies; you may hear that one in 12–14 women will get it. Remember that this is a *cumulative, lifetime* risk that is age-dependent. Younger women are much less likely to develop breast cancer, with the risk only slowly increasing with age.

My grandmother had breast cancer—will I get it too?

A number of factors will increase the risk of an individual developing breast cancer; some are rare but important (breast cancer susceptibility genes such as *BRCA1*) and others are more common but variable. Family history is important when it is a *first-degree* relative (sister, mother) and especially when the cancer was diagnosed pre-menopause or affected multiple relatives. With a relatively common disease such as breast cancer, having more distant relatives with breast cancer is usually just chance.

How is breast cancer managed?

Options for the diagnosis and treatment of breast cancer have expanded hugely over the last few years. Management in a multidisciplinary setting (with radiologists, surgeons, pathologists, oncologists, and reconstructive specialists) ensures the best outcomes for patients.

Answers

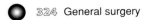

CASE 9.21 – 'I've found a breast lump.'

 Q1: What is the likely differential diagnosis?

A1

- Fibroadenoma

- Fat necrosis

- (Breast cancer—unlikely, but needs to be excluded).

 Q2: What issues in the given history support your final diagnosis?

A2

The age of the patient makes fibroadenoma the most likely diagnosis, with other benign lesions also possible. Breast cancer in this age group is extremely rare, but needs to be considered; a positive family history would increase one's concern.

Q3: What additional features in the history would you seek to support a particular diagnosis?

A3

Checking about trauma to the breast is useful, and may support a suspicion of fat necrosis.

Q4: What clinical examination would you perform and why?

A4

Clinical examination of both breasts (with a chaperone) should be performed. The axillary and supraclavicular nodal fields should be checked.

 Q5: What investigations would be most helpful and why?

A5

Investigations should be *imaging* and *pathology* to complete the 'triple assessment'. Mammography is difficult to interpret in the dense breasts of women under 35, and is usually not performed; ultrasound has greater diagnostic accuracy and is the imaging modality of choice in this group. Fine-needle aspiration cytology for a palpable lump is easily performed, and may be interpreted immediately by a pathologist in the clinic.

In this patient, clinical examination, ultrasound, and FNA are consistent and all support the diagnosis of fibroadenoma.

Q6: What treatment options are appropriate?

A6

The natural history of fibroadenomas is that about one third regress over time, one third remain the same, and one third continue to grow. Women should understand this in order to make treatment choices.

Non-operative. Some women are reassured by a benign diagnosis, and prefer to avoid an operation. To minimise the risk of the very rare false-negative diagnosis or missing a phyllodes tumour, most Breast Units would recommend obtaining either a second definitely-benign FNA at another time, or obtaining tissue for histology (rather than cytology) by a core biopsy, usually under ultrasound guidance.

Operative. Removal of the fibroadenoma is usually possible with a small scar, often placed along the areolar margin for cosmetic reasons. This both confirms the diagnosis and treats the problem definitively.

 CASE 9.22 – 'Something has shown up on my screening mammogram.'

 Q1: What is the likely differential diagnosis?

A1

Flecks of calcium on mammograms are reasonably common, and their likely diagnosis depends on their shape, size, and number. Large calcifications are usually not associated with cancer, and some configurations of calcium deposition may be pathognomonic, such as cup-shaped dependent calcium in cysts. In contrast, groups of small calcifications ('clustered microcalcifications') may be associated with extra breast cell activity, usually benign, but sometimes in areas of early cancer or DCIS.

 Q2: What issues in the given history support your final diagnosis?

A2

The *lack* of family history, or the presence of a lump, is now the most common presentation of breast cancer—screening mammography is intended to identify breast cancer or DCIS *early* to allow earlier treatment. (Large studies have now shown this is effective on a population basis, and most developed countries now have a screening program).

 Q3: What additional features in the history would you seek to support a particular diagnosis?

A3

Family history should again be determined for both breast and ovarian carcinoma; although useless to the patient herself, this may have implications for her children if positive.

Q4: What clinical examination would you perform and why?

A4

Breast examination is required, along with complete physical examination.

 Q5: What investigations would be most helpful and why?

A5

The screening mammogram should be reviewed, and sometimes further imaging workup (mammography and ultrasound) is required. Any previous screening films should also be reviewed and audited to assess if the lesion was identifiable earlier. As the lesion is not palpable, a mammographic or ultrasound guided stereotactic core biopsy should be obtained.

Subsequent histology of the stereotactic core biopsy shows ductal carcinoma in situ (DCIS).

 Q6: What treatment options are appropriate?

A6

Treatment options for DCIS are wide local excision (WLE) if well-localized, or mastectomy if covering a large area or multi-focal. To aid excision of an impalpable lesion, a wire is placed with the tip adjacent to the area needing removal. Axillary node dissection (AND) is not performed for *in-situ* disease due to the minimal risk of nodal spread. DCIS may widely ramify in the breast, so surgical margins need to be thoroughly examined to ensure clearance. Further excisions may be required to obtain this. In high-grade or extensive DCIS there is evidence that radiotherapy reduces the rate of local recurrence. Half of all recurrences will be invasive so it is vital to perform optimal treatment. Immediate reconstruction should be offered to any woman undergoing a mastectomy.

 CASE 9.23 – 'I've found a lump under my armpit.'

 Q1: What is the likely differential diagnosis?

A1

Diagnosis is secure, but attention should be directed to the presence of any symptoms suggestive of distant metastatic spread.

Q2: What issues in the given history support your final diagnosis?

A2

See above

Q3: What additional features in the history would you seek to support a particular diagnosis?

A3

See above

 Q4: What clinical examination would you perform and why?

A4

Complete physical examination should search for metastases.

 Q5: What investigations would be most helpful and why?

A5

Investigations should focus on staging the disease, and determining risk factors for anaesthesia.

 Q6: What treatment options are appropriate?

A6

Unless the patient chooses a non-operative approach, surgery is required and is often supplemented by radiotherapy, chemotherapy, hormonal manipulation, or a combination of these. In a women presenting with proven nodal disease and a tumour unsuitable for WLE, chemotherapy can be given prior to surgery (neo-adjuvant treatment). This has the benefit of reducing the size of the tumour, allowing breast-conserving surgery and also demonstrating the efficacy of the chemotherapy. In patients with extensive co-morbidities, that prevent surgical treatment, neo-adjuvant endocrine treatment can be used.

Surgical. The operation is performed for local control of disease, and to obtain prognostic information about the tumour that may tailor subsequent treatment. The main choice to be made is between WLE (with radiotherapy to the remaining breast) and mastectomy, either of which are accompanied by axillary node dissection. *These offer equivalent survival outcomes, and should usually be the choice of the patient.* Reconstructive surgery should ideally be offered to the patient considering mastectomy, and options include immediate or delayed reconstruction, and the use of implants or endogenous tissue (such as the transverse rectus abdominus myocutaneous (TRAM) flap or the latissimus dorsi flap). Axillary dissection is undergoing re-evaluation, and many units are now studying whether a sentinel node biopsy (SNB) may provide adequate staging information without the morbidity of completely removing the lymph nodes under the arm, which has a degree of morbidity. This is not appropriate in a woman with proven nodal disease.

Radiotherapy is used where wide local excision (WLE) is performed, but may also be offered for aggressive tumours. This may be directed to the chest wall, axilla and supraclavicular regions.

Chemotherapy is offered for aggressive tumours to reduce the risk of metastatic disease. Patients with positive lymph nodes are usually considered for chemotherapy, but node-negative patients with large, high-grade tumours, or younger patients, also benefit.

Hormonal manipulation is given in patients who have hormonally sensitive tumours (oestrogen and/or progesterone receptor positive). Tamoxifen (which binds to the oestrogen receptor) has been joined by the aromatase-inhibitor group of drugs (preventing androgens being coverted to oestrodiol). These greatly reduce cancer recurrence and are well tolerated.

♟♟ OSCE Counselling Cases – Answers

OSCE COUNSELLING CASE 9.11 – 'What can I do for this breast pain?'

Breast pain is surprisingly common amongst women. It may be *cyclical* or *non-cyclical*, and a careful history will determine the timing and any trigger factors. After history and examination has excluded any other aetiology, options for breast pain can be discussed. Most women will cope with the discomfort on being reassured there is nothing sinister causing the pain.

The importance of a correctly-fitted bra should be emphasised, and specialised sports bras may be useful for periods of vigorous exercise. The two most important avoidable factors in true breast pain are smoking and caffeine intake, and a breast pain presentation is a valuable opportunity to reinforce smoking cessation advice.

Simple analgesics may be appropriate if the pain is pronounced only during part of the menstrual cycle. Some women find Evening Primrose Oil useful—this needs to be taken in moderately high doses and for a prolonged period before the peak benefit is obtained, but has very few side effects and does not require a prescription.

OSCE COUNSELLING CASE 9.12 – 'I'm confused by my surgical options for breast cancer. Which should I choose?'

For most women (except those with very advanced tumours), it has been determined by a number of well-performed studies that breast-conserving surgery—i.e. Wide local excision (WLE) followed by radiotherapy to the remaining breast—results in equivalent overall survival to mastectomy, and a similar incidence of local recurrence. Accordingly, the choice of operation should be the patient's. Whatever approach is used, it should be made clear to the woman that she will be supported with as much information as she feels is needed to make a decision.

Many women feel that time is critical, and they want to have their operation as soon as possible. It is worth emphasising that breast cancer is usually a slowly growing tumour, and by diagnosis it may have been present for many months or even years. Allowing some days or a week or two to make a decision will not jeopardise the outcome, but may allow un-pressured choices to be made.

Mastectomy has a major impact on the body image of most women. For women who choose mastectomy (or for whom WLE is not appropriate for some reason), reconstructive surgery should usually be discussed and offered. Very rarely, resource constraints limit choices—if either radiotherapy or reconstructive surgery is available, mastectomy remains an excellent operation from the cancer point of view, but this is clearly suboptimal in the overall care of the patient.

Axillary node staging gives prognostic information that influences adjuvant treatment . *Sentinel lymph node biopsy* is a technique of identifying the first node that drains the breast. This is performed using a blue dye and radio-active colloid. This has the significant benefit of reduce post-operative morbidity when compared to axillary node clearance or sampling. If this node is clear the presumption is there has been no spread to the axillary nodes. Unfortunately its sensitivity is not 100 per cent, plus if the node is positive it usually requires a full axillary block dissection or axillary radiotherapy.

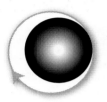

Index